W9-CCR-896

Seven Guidelines for Heart-Healthy Nutrition

- Choose a variety of fruits and vegetables daily — at least five servings.
- Choose a variety of whole grain foods daily.
- Choose healthy fats in moderation and limit your intake of saturated fat and transfat.
- Use less salt and choose prepared foods with less salt.
- Choose beverages and foods to moderate your intake of sugar.
- If you consume alcohol, do so in moderation.
- Do not consume more calories than are required to maintain your best body weight.

Major Risk Factors for Coronary Artery Disease

- High blood pressure
- Elevated cholesterol
- Cigarette smoking
- Inactive lifestyle
- Obesity
- Diabetes

Five Keys to Staying with Your Physical Activity Program

- **Set a time and place.** Plan at least one activity like a short walk at lunch, and other opportunities will fall in place.
- **Be prepared.** Adopt a mind-set that emphasizes more physical activity.
- **Include family and friends.**
- **Have fun.** You'll stick with something you like.
- **Prioritize.** Make getting physical activity as important a priority as other objectives in your life.

Tips for Lowering Stress

- **Modify factors that can compound stress.** Get enough rest. Don't overconsume caffeine. And so on.
- **Live in the present.** Quit fearing the future or regretting the past. Make the most of today.
- **Get out of your own way.** Don't dwell on the negative or indulge in negative self-talk.
- **Take time out.** Step away from it all for ten minutes a day. Take a stroll. Meditate. Nap. Tune into the calm.

For Dummies: Bestselling Book Series for Beginners

Heart Disease For Dummies®

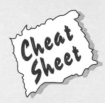
Cheat Sheet

Warning Signs of Heart Attack

Even if you've never had a single sign of trouble, call 911 and go straight to the hospital for prompt evaluation if you experience any of these warning signs of heart attack.

- Uncomfortable pressure, fullness, squeezing, or pain in the center of the chest lasting more than a few minutes
- Pain spreading to the shoulders, neck, or arms
- Chest discomfort with lightheadedness, fainting, sweating, nausea, or shortness of breath

Questions to Ask the Doctor

When you're being evaluated for heart disease or any other condition, asking these questions can help you get the information you need.

- What's my diagnosis?
- What tests will I need to undergo?
- Do these tests have any side effects or dangers?
- What's the recommended treatment?
- What are the potential side effects of the treatment?
- What treatment choices are available?
- Should I be asking any other questions?
- Is there any source of information that I can read about my diagnosis?

Keys to Modifying Your Risk Factors for Heart Disease

- Control high blood pressure. Optimal blood pressure is 120/80 mm Hg or below.
- Control your cholesterol levels. Desirable levels are below 200 mg/dl. The lower the better.
- Accumulate at least 30 minutes of moderate physical activity on most, if not all, days.
- Maintain your body weight at healthy levels — a body mass index between 19 and 25.
- If you smoke, quit.

For Dummies: Bestselling Book Series for Beginners

Heart Disease

FOR

DUMMIES®

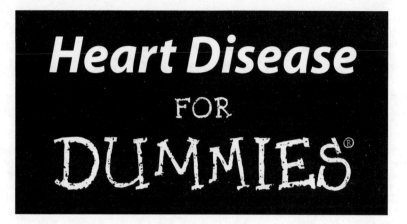

Heart Disease FOR DUMMIES®

by James M. Rippe, MD
Founder and director of the Center for Clinical
and Lifestyle Research

Associate Professor of Cardiology, Tufts University

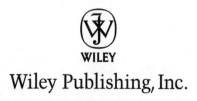

WILEY

Wiley Publishing, Inc.

Heart Disease For Dummies®

Published by
Wiley Publishing, Inc.
111 River St.
Hoboken, NJ 07030-5774
www.wiley.com

For general information on our other products and services or to obtain technical support, please contact our Customer Care Department within the U.S. at 800-762-2974, outside the U.S. at 317-572-3993, or fax 317-572-4002.

Wiley also publishes its books in a variety of electronic formats. Some content that appears in print may not be available in electronic books.

Library of Congress Control Number: 2004100891

ISBN: 0-7645-4155-2

Manufactured in the United States of America

1O/QW/QS/QU/IN

About the Author

Dr. Rippe is a graduate of Harvard College and Harvard Medical School with postgraduate training at Massachusetts General Hospital. He is the founder and director of the Center for Clinical and Lifestyle Research and Associate Professor of Medicine (Cardiology) at Tufts University School of Medicine.

Dr. Rippe is founder and director of the Rippe Health Assessment at Florida Hospital Celebration Health. This is a series of comprehensive health evaluations for high-performance individuals conducted at the state-of-the-art medical and fitness facility of Celebration Health in Orlando, Florida.

Dr. Rippe is regarded as one of the leading authorities on preventive cardiology, health and fitness, and healthy weight loss in the United States. Under his leadership, the Rippe Lifestyle Institute has conducted numerous research projects on cardiovascular risk-factor reduction, fitness walking, weight loss, running, basketball, bodybuilding, cycling, rowing, cholesterol reduction, and low-fat diets. Laboratory members have presented more than 120 papers at national, medical, and scientific meetings in the last ten years. Dr. Rippe has written more than 200 publications on issues in medicine, health and fitness, and weight management. He has also written or edited 30 books, including 18 medical texts and 12 books on health and fitness for the general public, including *Fitness Walking* (Perigee, 1985), *The Sports Performance Factors* (Perigee, 1986), and *Fitness Walking for Women* (Perigee, 1987). Both walking books were recipients of National American Health Book Awards. His book on executive fitness, *Fit for Success,* was published by Prentice Hall Press in June 1989. His book on walking and weight loss, *The Rockport Walking Program,* was published in fall 1989. Another one of his books, *The Complete Book of Fitness Walking,* was published by Prentice Hall Press in June 1990. His book, *The Exercise Exchange Program,* combining exercise and proper nutrition, was published in February 1992. *Fit Over Forty,* published in 1996, explores lifestyle issues related to cardiovascular health, particularly for individuals older than 40, and focuses on motivating people to take simple steps to take charge of their health and lives. *The Joint Pain Prescription,* published in 2001, gives practical advice about preventing arthritis.

Dr. Rippe also edits a major textbook that teaches physicians about diverse aspects of cardiovascular medicine and the impact of lifestyle decisions on good health. This textbook, *Lifestyle Medicine* (Blackwell Science, 1999), is the first textbook to guide physicians in the diverse aspects of how to incorporate lifestyle recommendations into the practice of modern medicine. His intensive-care textbook, *Irwin and Rippe's Intensive Care Medicine* (5th edition, 2003; co-edited with Dr. Richard Irwin), is the world's leading textbook on intensive and coronary care.

Dr. Rippe has developed corporate fitness programs for a variety of companies, including Allstate Life Insurance and The Shimizu Corporation. He serves as Chairman of the Advisory Board for the "Healthy Growing Up" program — a curriculum linking health and fitness for children that was made available free of charge to every U.S. school system in 1992.

Dr. Rippe's work has been featured on *The Today Show, Good Morning America*, PBS's "BodyWatch," CBS Morning and Evening News, CNN, and in a variety of print media, including *The New York Times, New York Times Magazine, L.A. Times, The Wall Street Journal*, and many monthly publications. He comments regularly on health and fitness for *USA Today, American Health,* and *Prevention.* He served for three years as medical editor for the Television Food Network (TVFN).

In 1989, Dr. Rippe was named Fitness Educator of the Year by the International Dance Exercise Association (IDEA). In 1990, he was named one of the 10 national "Healthy American Fitness Leaders" by the United States Jaycees and the President's Council on Physical Fitness and Sports. In 1992, he received a Lifetime Achievement Award from IDEA.

A lifelong and avid athlete, Dr. Rippe maintains his personal fitness with a regular walk, jog, and weight-training program. He holds a black belt in karate and is an avid windsurfer, skier, and tennis player. He lives outside of Boston with his wife, television news anchor Stephanie Hart, and their four children, Hart, Jaelin, Devon, and Jamie.

Dedication

To Stephanie, Hart, Jaelin, Devon, and Jamie, who make my heart sing and provide the cornerstone for my personal program to maintain a healthy heart.

Author's Acknowledgments

It would be impossible to cite all of the individuals who have provided advice and support during the time it took to complete this book. However, several deserve special recognition for their significant contributions.

First, I would like to acknowledge and applaud the superb writing and editorial skills of my main collaborator, Mary Abbott Waite. This is the sixth book project on which Mary Abbott and I have collaborated. Mary Abbott is a dream writing partner. She has taken complex medical topics and edited my thoughts in a way that makes the message clear, concise, and user-friendly (and, we hope, at times even a little humorous!). Mary Abbott not only writes well but also is a superb researcher. She verified a number of topics that I introduced in various chapters by performing considerable outside research from a variety of other expert sources. She has often added interesting and helpful tips and anecdotes that come either from her own experience or from her friends and relatives.

Second, my Editorial Director and good friend, Beth Porcaro, applied her formidable organization skills to keep this whole process moving forward and on time. Beth manages to accomplish an unbelievable amount of work while maintaining great judgment and a wonderful sense of humor.

I also would like to commend and thank top chefs from across America who wrote the recipes that are included in this book. These include: MaryAnn Saporito Boothroyd, Garrett Cho, Alfonso Constriciani, Constantin Kerageorgiou, Frank McClelland, Donna Nordin, Walter Pisano, Nora Pouillon, Mark Tarbell, and Carl Walker. Titles, restaurant names, and restaurant locations for the contributing chefs can be found with their recipes.

I am also indebted to the talented research staff at my laboratory, the Rippe Lifestyle Institute in Shrewsbury, Massachusetts, and Celebration, Florida. Under the superb direction of Research Director Ted Angelopoulos, PhD, MPH, our staff of health-care and research professionals manages to keep a busy laboratory humming along while freeing up time for me to tackle major writing projects such as this.

Many of the clinical insights from this book are employed on a daily basis at my clinical facility, the Rippe Health Assessment at Florida Hospital Celebration Health. My superb staff there have all provided useful insights and ongoing clinical validation of many of the concepts discussed in this book.

My professional colleagues have been a source of continuing intellectual stimulation throughout my career as a cardiologist. I would like to particularly acknowledge Dr. Joseph Alpert, Chief of Medicine at the University of Arizona, who was an early mentor at Harvard Medical School and who has continued to support and fuel my interest in preventive cardiology. Dr. Ira Ockene, Professor of Medicine and Director of the Preventive Cardiology program at UMass Medical School, was an early mentor in invasive cardiology and coronary care and has continued to help clarify my thinking in all aspects of preventive cardiology. My friend and colleague Dr. Richard Irwin has taught me a great deal about both the practice of medicine and the writing and editing of books.

My responsibilities and commitments as a cardiologist and researcher, teacher, consultant, and writer require meticulous attention to details and schedules. My executive assistant, Carol Moreau, does an almost miraculous job in keeping all of these strands of my life intertwined with considerable grace and competence and never loses her cool.

Last, but certainly not least, my darling wife, Stephanie Hart Rippe, has provided the safe harbor without which none of these voyages, literary or otherwise, would be conceivable. While supporting my intense work schedule and often outlandish travel arrangements, she has grounded me with her love and inspired me with her courage, beauty, and intelligence. In addition, she has given me four beautiful daughters: Hart Elizabeth Rippe, Jaelin Davis Rippe, Devon Marshall Rippe, and Jamie Conrad Rippe. These five individuals, who together comprise the "Rippe Women," continue to make it all worthwhile and have convinced me that I'm not only the luckiest but also the most-loved man in the universe.

To all of these individuals and many others who have helped along the way, my heartfelt gratitude. I hope the final product reflects the strength, commitment, and caring of all those who made it possible. In a small way, I hope that this book helps people who are either engaged in an ongoing battle against the number-one killer in our country — heart disease — or who are seeking to prevent it by providing useful facts, information, and above all motivation to live a heart-healthy lifestyle.

Publisher's Acknowledgments

We're proud of this book; please send us your comments through our Dummies online registration form located at www.dummies.com/register/.

Some of the people who helped bring this book to market include the following:

Acquisitions, Editorial, and Media Development

Project Editor: Traci Cumbay

Acquisitions Editor: Natasha Graf

Copy Editor: E. Neil Johnson

Assistant Editor: Holly Grimes

Technical Editor: Julia H. Indik, MD, PhD

Senior Permissions Editor: Carmen Krikorian

Editorial Manager: Jennifer Ehrlich

Editorial Assistant: Elizabeth Rea

Cover Photos: ©Michael Pole/CORBIS

Cartoons: Rich Tennant, www.the5thwave.com

Production

Project Coordinator: Courtney MacIntyre

Layout and Graphics: Andrea Dahl, Lauren Goodard, Joyce Haughey, Heather Ryan, Jacque Schneider

Proofreaders: Laura Albert, Andy Hollandbeck, Carl William Pierce, TECHBOOKS Production Services

Indexer: TECHBOOKS Production Services

Publishing and Editorial for Consumer Dummies

Diane Graves Steele, Vice President and Publisher, Consumer Dummies

Joyce Pepple, Acquisitions Director, Consumer Dummies

Kristin A. Cocks, Product Development Director, Consumer Dummies

Michael Spring, Vice President and Publisher, Travel

Brice Gosnell, Associate Publisher, Travel

Kelly Regan, Editorial Director, Travel

Publishing for Technology Dummies

Andy Cummings, Vice President and Publisher, Dummies Technology/General User

Composition Services

Gerry Fahey, Vice President of Production Services

Debbie Stailey, Director of Composition Services

Contents at a Glance

Table of Contents

Introduction

. . . .

Consider these facts:

✔ One American dies of heart disease every 33 seconds — amounting to almost one million deaths every year.

✔ Almost one in four Americans has one or more types of heart disease.

✔ Considering all risk factors for heart disease — high blood pressure, high cholesterol, smoking, being overweight, physical inactivity — not one family in America is left untouched by heart disease.

✔ Regardless of your age, sex, ethnicity, and current heart health, you can acquire the knowledge and take action to work toward a healthier heart and the benefits that go with it.

As you hold this book in your hand to read these facts, your heart is beating away in your chest, sustaining your life. Although it's about the size of a clenched adult fist and weighs less than a pound, your heart beats 40 million times a year and generates enough force to lift you 100 miles into the atmosphere. What an amazing — and absolutely essential — machine!

Why This Book?

Heart Disease For Dummies is a common-sense guide for everyone. In this book, I give you some advice, simple diagrams, and yes, even an occasional stern lecture about simple things that you can do every day to maximize your cardiac function. You'll also find some basic strategies and lifestyle practices to reduce your risk of the major forms of heart disease.

If you (or your loved ones) already have heart disease or if you want to lower your risk of getting it, you have come to the right place. I run the largest exercise, nutrition, and cardiac lifestyle research laboratory in the world. I am also a board-certified cardiologist and editor of the major intensive-care textbook in the United States. I personally have performed thousands of heart catheterizations and taken care of many people with all forms of heart disease. I rely on that background and the many important conversations that I've had with patients to give you some simple advice about the common conditions related to heart disease. I explore some facts related to coronary artery disease, angina, heart attacks, hypertension, heart failure, and many other cardiac conditions. Along the way, I hope to answer those questions that I am commonly asked and those I suspect many of my patients had but may have been afraid to ask.

When you were born, you were given one heart and one life. Making the best of both is up to you. This book's goal is to provide simple, straightforward information and answers to help you do just that.

How This Heart Owner's Manual Is Organized

"Begin at the beginning," instructs the King of Hearts in *Alice's Adventures in Wonderland.* That's sound advice, so here's how to get started.

Part 1: Understanding Heart Disease

Part I provides the basic information you need to understand how heart disease affects your heart and your life. Chapter 1 covers why you need to care more about your heart; Chapter 2 explains how the heart works; and Chapter 3 describes the conditions and activities that put the heart at risk for disease.

Part 11: Identifying the Many Forms of Heart Disease

Speaking of the dangers of the Great Depression, President Franklin Roosevelt observed, "The only thing we have to fear is fear itself." Fear of heart disease — that you either have it or may get it — can be immobilizing. Modern science and medicine offer many strategies to prevent, diagnose, control, and manage this public health enemy number one. As a heart owner, you'll find that knowledge is power. Each chapter in this section takes the mystery and fear out of the common conditions that can plague the heart and gives you the ammunition you need to fight back as you work in partnership with your physician and other medical allies.

Chapter 4 covers coronary artery disease, which is the leading cause of death from heart disease and is associated with a wide variety of serious syndromes including angina (chronic chest pain) and heart attack. Chapter 5 looks at heart attacks. Then I turn to other common conditions — rhythm disturbances in Chapter 6 and heart failure (as in congestive heart failure) in Chapter 7. Chapter 8 discusses stroke, a major form of cardiovascular disease and the third leading cause of death in the United States. Chapter 9 covers other cardiac conditions such as valvular heart disease, pericardial disease, and congenital abnormalities (conditions that some people are born with).

Part III: Finding Out Whether You Have Heart Disease

Physicians and modern medical science have extensive diagnostic techniques and tests to assess the state of your heart's health. In Chapter 10, I discuss how your doctor assesses your heart health and risk of heart disease in a checkup. Chapter 11 is a quick and friendly guide to all the tests and procedures used in evaluating heart problems. Chapter 12 tells you what you need to know about working with your doctor effectively.

Part IV: Controlling and Treating Heart Disease

Controlling health conditions that help cause heart disease is a big part of treating many manifestations of heart disease. Chapter 13 discusses controlling high blood pressure, and Chapter 14 deals with controlling cholesterol. Chapter 15 reviews the most common drug and medical treatments available for treating heart disease, and Chapter 16 covers invasive medical and surgical procedures. I explore alternative therapies in Chapter 17.

Part V: Living Well with Heart Disease

If you've had a heart attack or heart surgery, returning to health and a high quality of life starts with cardiac rehabilitation, which I cover in Chapter 18. Is heart disease ever reversible? I look at all the evidence in Chapter 19.

Modern science shows that simple strategies based on proper nutrition, physical activity, weight management, and mind/body connections can both prevent and help control heart disease. Chapter 20 offers compact guidelines for heart-healthy nutrition. Chapter 21 covers the whys, wherefores, and benefits of physical activity. Chapter 22 offers tips about drawing on the power of mind/body connections to reduce stress and achieve success. Chapter 23 provides resources to help you quit smoking, the most important step a smoker can take in improving heart health.

Part VI: The Part of Tens

Even if you skip the rest of the book and do nothing but memorize the ten tips in each of these four chapters, your heart will *still* thank you.

Oh, and go to the Appendix to check out ten of the tastiest and healthiest dishes ever set before mortal man and woman. If you think healthy eating, by its very nature, has to be boring, you underestimate some of America's leading chefs.

Icons Used in This Book

This icon signals physiological and scientific information about the heart. But don't worry — all technical stuff is presented in plain English.

You find facts, practices, and insights that promote or enhance heart health alongside this icon.

The fields of health, fitness, and medicine abound with ideas — some very popular — that have no basis in fact or that are outdated. When it ain't so, I say so.

This icon indicates practical suggestions you can put to work to help you reach your heart-health goals.

Think of this icon as a caution flag.

Part I
Understanding Heart Disease

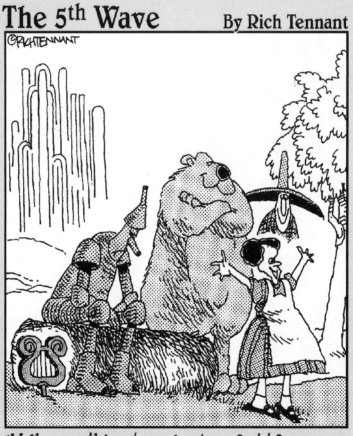

The 5th Wave   By Rich Tennant

"Well, everything turned out perfect! Scarecrow has a brain, the lion found his courage, and the Tin Man *got* a harp."

In this part . . .

Find the basic information you need to begin taking control of your heart health. First, I share with you why you need to understand how heart disease can affect your life and the good news of what you can do about it. Then it's time to explore how the miracle machine that is your heart works — cardiac anatomy covered painlessly in one easy chapter. Then I give you an overview of what behaviors and conditions increase your risk of developing heart disease and what you can do about them.

Chapter 1

Confronting Heart Disease: The No. 1 Health Threat

....

....

*W*hy is the heart so magical for us? Why do we tell our loved ones that they live inside our hearts? Why do we say that someone with enormous courage has "tremendous heart"? Why are lovers said to die of a broken heart? Everyone has an emotional attachment to this miraculous pump that is inconceivable for any other organ. Would you ever think about your lungs or kidneys or pancreas in this way? Of course not. Humans seem to have a built-in sense of the heart's importance. And cardiovascular disease in all its forms is the biggest threat to our hearts.

Exploring How Heart Disease Affects Your Life

The heart captivates our imagination for good reason — human health, daily performance, and life itself depend on the heart. The heart and the cardiovascular system have amazing sophistication, strength, and durability. At the same time, the health of the heart rests in a fragile balance. When even small parts of its complex machinery are a little bit out of whack, the heart can cause great discomfort, pain, and even death.

Despite the emotional energy we attach to our hearts and the heart's crucial importance to life itself, most people are pretty ignorant about the heart and how it works. You know you can't live without one. You know that heart disease is pretty common and more than a little scary. So when your doctor says your cholesterol levels or elevated blood pressure is raising your risk of heart disease, it's a little alarming. And the bottom falls out of your stomach if your physician says, "I don't think that chest pain is a muscle strain. We'd better do some tests to rule out heart disease." At moments like that you wish you knew more about that small pump thumping away in your chest and all the things that threaten it and what you can do about them. That's where *Heart Disease For Dummies* comes in.

Facing the bad news about heart disease

Heart disease is public health enemy number one in America. In one or another of its manifestations, heart disease touches virtually every family in the United States. Consider these startling facts:

- Almost 60 million Americans — almost one in every four — have one or more types of heart disease.

- Heart disease and stroke cause more than one of every two deaths — more deaths than all other diseases combined.

- An individual is more than 10 times more likely to die of heart disease than in an accident and more than 30 times as likely to die of heart disease than of AIDS.

- Heart disease is an equal-opportunity killer. It is the leading cause of death in men and women and all ethnic and racial groups in the United States.

- If money is the most important thing in your life, you might like to know that the yearly estimated cost of cardiovascular disease in the United States is $286.5 *billion*.

As a cardiologist, I've seen these statistics made all too real in the lives of too many patients. But I've also seen what people can do to take charge of heart health at all stages, from working to lower their risk of developing heart disease to learning how to control and live well with advanced coronary artery disease (CAD) and its varied manifestations.

Seizing the good news about preventing and controlling heart disease

The bad-news facts about heart disease are real, but they aren't the only news. Extensive research proves that you can do many things in your daily life and in working with your physician to use the latest medical science that can preserve and maximize the health of your heart — even if you already have heart disease. Consider these good-news facts:

- ✔ People who are physically active on a regular basis cut their risk of heart disease in half.

- ✔ People who stop smoking cigarettes can return their risk of heart disease and stroke to almost normal levels within five years after stopping.

- ✔ Overweight people who lose as little as 5 percent to 10 percent of their body weight can substantially lower their risk of heart disease.

- ✔ Simple changes in what you eat can lower blood cholesterol.

- ✔ The number of deaths from heart disease declined 20 percent during the last decade — a decline largely based on lifestyle changes.

Working with your physician to control heart disease

Even if you have CAD or have had a heart attack, clinical research shows that working with your physician in a supervised program to reduce your risk factors for heart disease is highly beneficial and even life saving. Take a look at what research reveals about how you can improve your health:

- ✔ If you have CAD, modifying risk factors such as high blood pressure, high blood cholesterol, physical inactivity, and being overweight can reduce your risk of a future heart attack or the need for coronary artery bypass surgery, and add years to your life.

- ✔ In clinical studies, people who experienced a heart attack or unstable angina and who lowered their total cholesterol by 18 percent and LDL cholesterol by 25 percent experienced a 24 percent decrease in death from cardiovascular disease when compared to a control group. The need for bypass surgery was reduced by 20 percent.

✔ Appropriate physical activity or exercise improves the ability to perform activities comfortably for people with angina and people who've had heart attacks or even coronary surgery.

✔ Weight loss can help lower cholesterol levels and control blood pressure and diabetes — conditions that contribute to the continued progress of heart disease.

✔ If you smoke and have had a heart attack, quitting smoking significantly reduces your risk of having a second heart attack or experiencing sudden death.

Checking Out Why You Should Care about Heart Disease

So who should care about heart disease? As the good news in the previous section proves, everyone. No matter your present state of heart health, you can do plenty to reduce your risk factors for heart disease. (Find out more about that in Chapter 3.) Young or old, man or woman, totally healthy or coping with heart disease or other health problems, regardless of ethnic and racial backgrounds, you need to care about heart disease. If you belong to certain groups, however, some associated facts and conditions should raise your consciousness about why paying attention to heart disease and heart health should be important to you.

Caring about heart disease, if you're a woman

Although heart disease is an equal-opportunity killer, many people, men and women alike, continue to think that heart disease is primarily a *man's* problem. Wrong! Consider these facts:

✔ More women than men die of heart disease in the United States.

✔ Although men suffer heart attacks an average of ten years earlier than women, after menopause women catch up. Within the year after a heart attack, 42 percent of women will die, compared to 24 percent of men.

✔ Women are less likely to know the warning signs for a heart attack.

✔ Women smokers are at six times greater risk of heart attack than non-smoking women.

✔ Amazingly, recent surveys show that women are more afraid of breast cancer than cardiovascular disease. Although without question breast cancer is a serious disease, only 1 woman in 27 dies from breast cancer, but 1 in 2 dies from heart disease.

In the final analysis, heart disease is at least as dangerous for women as it is for men.

So, if you're a woman who bought this book for the man in your life, think again. Keep this copy for yourself and buy another one for him! There is just as much in this book for you as there is for the men in your life.

Caring about heart disease, if you're African American

Heart disease is the leading cause of death for African Americans, just as it is for all Americans. Although every individual is different, African Americans, as a group, experience a higher incidence of certain conditions that contribute to the risk of heart disease. African Americans:

✔ Develop high blood pressure at earlier ages than White Americans, and at any decade of life, more have high blood pressure, which is a risk factor for heart disease and stroke

✔ Are 2.5 times more likely to die from stroke than European Americans

✔ Are twice as likely as non-Hispanic Whites to have diabetes, a factor that contributes to developing heart disease

Although heart disease is a leading cause of death for all women, Black women ages 35 to 74 have a death rate from heart disease that's nearly 72 percent higher than White women.

Although much current research seeks to determine the causes of the higher incidence of high blood pressure among African Americans, African Americans can prevent and control hypertension and other risk factors by adopting appropriate lifestyle practices.

Caring about heart disease, if you're a parent

The incidence of heart disease is, of course, very rare among children and youths. But the roots of heart disease are firmly planted in childhood. As people in the United States have spent more and more time in front of the TV or computer screen, commuting in cars, and eating out, children in the U.S. are learning lifestyle behaviors and developing health conditions that may make them more, rather than less, likely to develop heart disease and other health problems. The good (and bad) habits of a lifetime usually begin in childhood. Parents need to set good examples for their children and encourage them to adopt practices that optimize their future health. Consider the following facts about children in the U.S.:

- ✔ An estimated 4.1 million teenagers ages 12 to 17 smoke. More than 43 percent of high school students use tobacco products, and that percentage continues to grow. Smoking is a major contributor to heart disease, cancer, and other health problems.

- ✔ Approximately 50 percent of American teenagers get no regular physical activity.

- ✔ More than one in five children and youths, ages 6 to 17, are overweight, another risk factor for heart disease.

Caring about heart disease, if you're older

Unfortunately, many Americans expect heart trouble to be part of their older years. That need not be so. And if you *are* older and, for that matter, even if you already have heart disease, you can do plenty to avoid being part of these statistics:

- ✔ Approximately 84 percent of deaths from heart disease occur in people older than 65.

- ✔ People older than 65 account for about 85 percent of deaths from heart attack.

- ✔ After age 55, the incidence of stroke doubles with each decade of life.

- ✔ The most frequent cause of hospitalization for people older than 65 is congestive heart failure.

- ✔ In America, the older you get, the fatter you get. Americans are twice as likely to be overweight — a risk for heart disease they absolutely can control — at 65 than they were at 35.

Taking Charge of Your Heart Health

Without question, heart disease is a serious enemy. In fact, it's the biggest enemy. But, it's equally true that you can take charge of your heart health, whatever its present state.

As I often like to say: *Ipsa scientia potestas est,* or knowledge is power. (That Latin should get you ready for some of the medical terms I must occasionally use. Besides, I'm a doctor, so what did you expect?) The rest of *Heart Disease For Dummies* is full of information that can empower you to

✔ Understand the basics about heart health and heart disease

✔ Partner with your physician in putting the power of simple lifestyle practices and medical technology to work for you

Assessing Your Risk of a First Heart Attack

The statistics and facts that I share earlier in this chapter may have you thinking about your own risk of heart disease. Many tests help people assess their risk of developing CAD, in general, and first heart attacks, in particular. Based on data from the Framingham Heart Study, the longest and largest population study of heart disease, the test that follows helps you assess your risk of having a first heart attack, gives you a good idea of how you can modify your risk factors, and may highlight topics for you to talk about with your physician at your next checkup. You do have a regular checkup scheduled, don't you?

First Heart Attack Risk Test

This test can help you figure out your risk of having a first heart attack. Fill in your points for each risk factor. Then total them to find out your level of risk.

_____**Age (in years) Men:** Younger than 35, 0 points; 35 to 39, 1 point; 40 to 48, 2 points; 49 to 53, 3 points; and 54 and older, 4 points.

_____**Age (in years) Women:** Younger than 42, 0 points; 42 to 44, 1 point; 45 to 54, 2 points; 55 to 73, 3 points; 74 and older, 4 points.

_____**Family History:** A family history of heart disease or heart attacks before age 60 — 2 points.

_____**Inactive Lifestyle:** I rarely exercise or do anything physically demanding — 1 point.

_____**Weight:** I weigh 20 (or more) pounds more than my ideal weight — 1point.

_____**Smoking:** I'm a smoker — 1 point.

_____**Diabetic:** Male diabetic, 1 point; female diabetic, 2 points.

_____**Total Cholesterol Level:** Less than 240 mg/dl, 0 points; 240 to 315 mg/dl, 1 point; more than 315 mg/dl, 2 points.

_____**HDL Level (good cholesterol):** 35 to 59mg/dl, 0 points; 30 to 38 mg/dl, 1 point; less than 30 mg/dl, 2 points; more than 60 mg/dl, 1 point.

_____**Blood Pressure:** I don't take blood pressure medication; my blood pressure is _(use your top or higher blood pressure number)_: Less than 140 mmHg, 0 points; 140 to 170 mmHg, 1 point; greater than 170 mmHg, 2 points; or, I'm currently taking blood pressure medication — 1 point.

_____**Total Points**

If you scored 4 points or more, you may be above the average risk of a first heart attack compared to the general adult population. The more points you score, the higher your risk. (Based on data from The Framingham Study, as adapted by Bristol Meyer Squib.)

If you scored 4 points or more and haven't had a recent checkup, scheduling one soon is a good idea. You may also want to take your risk assessment results in to discuss with your physician.

Benefiting from heart health

Taking control of your heart health offers other wonderful upsides for living well that include

✔ **Improving your overall health:** Many of the steps that benefit your heart health also improve your total health and fitness, to say nothing of your good looks.

✔ **Increasing functionality:** Use it or lose it, goes the old saying. The healthier your heart, the greater the probability that you can stay active, mobile, and engaged in pursuits that interest you for a long, long time.

✔ **Increasing economic benefits:** The healthier you are, the lower your health-care costs, and the more money in your pocket for fun things.

✔ **Increasing longevity:** Keeping your heart healthy is not an iron-clad guarantee that you'll live longer, but considering the mortality rates of people with heart disease (reviewed earlier in this chapter), even card-carrying "Dummies" can figure out that keeping your heart as healthy as possible can keep the grim reaper away longer.

✔ **Having more fun:** Nothing slows you down or scares the family like a heart attack. Angina pain, angioplasty, coronary artery bypass surgery, and other common outcomes of heart disease aren't picnics in the park, either. Working for heart health and controlling heart disease can help you avoid these problems.

Chapter 2

Touring the Heart and Cardiovascular System

*Y*our heart, my heart, every human heart . . . Figure 2-1 shows pretty much what each looks like. Not much to look at, is it? The average adult heart is about the size of a clenched fist and weighs less than a pound. But your life depends on your heart. The heart is the *engine* that keeps your body functioning. When disease or injury strikes the heart, the body's ability to function declines as the heart's ability declines.

In this chapter, I discuss how your heart and cardiovascular system are structured — their anatomy and how they accomplish their amazing work. A sound knowledge of the anatomy of your heart helps you better understand the many forms of heart disease I discuss in later chapters. This knowledge also enhances your understanding of the varied therapies and procedures used to treat varied forms of heart disease.

Can you skip this chapter? Sure, but I wouldn't. Even if you begin hyperventilating (or snoozing) at the mere idea of technical stuff, don't forget that knowledge is power. You'll be glad you got a grip on these basics. They help you be a better partner in your healthcare.

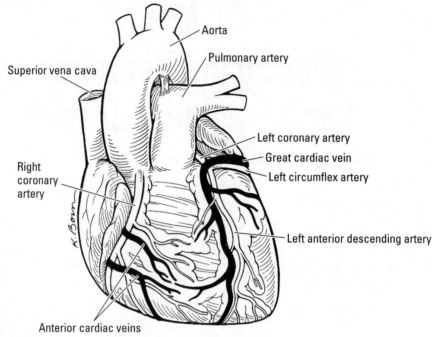

Aorta

Pulmonary artery

Superior vena cava

Left coronary artery

Great cardiac vein

Left circumflex artery

Right coronary artery

Left anterior descending artery

Figure 2-1:
A typical healthy heart.

Anterior cardiac veins

Pumping for Life: The Heart

The heart is located in the center of the chest cavity. About one-third rests beneath the breastbone, or *sternum,* and two-thirds rest to the left of the midline of the body. The breastbone, rib cage, muscles, and other structures of the chest wall protect the heart. In the average adult, the heart pumps 5 quarts of blood per minute at rest and 25 to 30 quarts per minute at maximum effort. In highly trained athletes working at maximum effort, the amount of blood pumped per minute can run as high as 40 quarts.

The heart muscle

The walls of the heart are made up of a unique muscle called the myocardium (*myo* = muscle and *cardium* = heart; pronounced my-o-*car*-dee-um). This muscle is the only one of its kind in the body because it must be supplied with oxygenated blood at all times to survive. By contrast, other muscles, such as those of the arms and legs, although still highly dependent on oxygenated blood, can perform briefly in the absence of oxygen (as when you dash from your car to the store during a rainshower). The heart is denied this luxury. For the heart to keep beating, arteries that feed the heart, the *coronary arteries,* must deliver a continuous supply of oxygenated blood. That's why the narrowing of these arteries, which is known as *coronary artery disease (CAD),* is so dangerous to the heart. When the coronary arteries grow narrower, a series of adverse events ensues, starting with *angina* (*an*-juh-nuh), or chest pain (Chapter 4), and ranging all the way to heart attack (Chapter 5) and, potentially, sudden death (Chapter 5).

The heart as a pump

The heart is a magnificent four-chambered pump that has two jobs:

- ✓ Pumping blood to the lungs to get oxygen
- ✓ Pumping the oxygenated blood to the rest of the body

To fulfill these tasks, the heart has a left and a right side (as shown in Figure 2-2), each with one main pumping chamber called a *ventricle* located in the lower part of it. Sitting above the left and right ventricles are two small booster pumps called *atria* (or *atrium,* when you're talking about just one). The right ventricle pumps deoxygenated blood, which returns from the body through veins and the right atrium, out into the lungs where it receives a new supply of oxygen. The blood then returns to the heart, first entering the left atrium and then the left ventricle. The left ventricle pumps oxygenated blood through the arterial system out to the rest of the body where it feeds every vital organ — in fact, every single living cell you have.

A thick muscular wall called the *septum* separates the left and right ventricles. Valves regulate the flow of blood in and out of the heart and from chamber to chamber. Various disease conditions can damage each of these structures.

The heart valves

The heart has four valves that act a bit like cardiac traffic cops by directing the way blood flows, how much of it flows, and when to stop it from flowing. Take a look at the positions of the four valves (defined in the list that follows) and how they direct blood flow through the heart, as illustrated in Figure 2-3.

- ✓ The *tricuspid* (try-*cuhs*-pid) valve, so called because it has three cusps, or flaps, opens to enable blood to flow into the right ventricle when the heart is relaxed and closes when the heart contracts to prevent blood from going back into the body.

✔ The *mitral* valve (*my*-trul), which resembles a bishop's miter (hat), controls the blood flow between the left atrium and the left ventricle. (The next time you see the Pope in full regalia, think of his hat as resembling the structure of a mitral valve in the heart.)

✔ The *pulmonic* (pull-*mon*-ik) valve controls the flow of blood from the right ventrical to the pulmonary artery supplying the lungs. (This valve is called *pulmonic* because the Latin word for lungs is the root word for *pulmonary.*)

✔ The *aortic* (ay-*or*-tik) valve, which separates the left ventricle from the aorta, opens to enable blood flow to the body when the heart contracts and closes when the heart relaxes to prevent blood from flowing back into the heart.

Disease and injury can cause heart valves to leak, narrow, or otherwise malfunction, disrupting the heart's ability to pump blood efficiently. (I discuss valve problems in Chapter 9.)

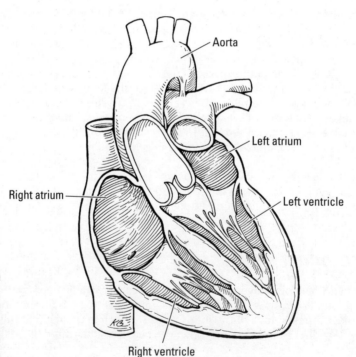

Figure 2-2:
The four chambers of the heart.

Aorta

Left atrium

Right atrium

Left ventricle

Right ventricle

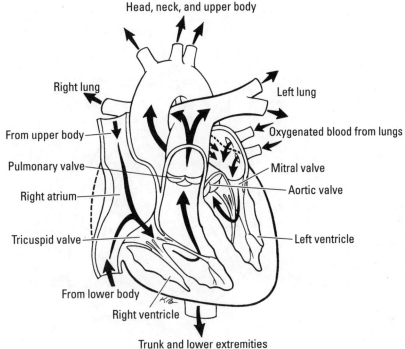

Head, neck, and upper body

Right lung

Left lung

From upper body

Oxygenated blood from lungs

Pulmonary valve

Mitral valve

Right atrium

Aortic valve

Tricuspid valve

Left ventricle

Figure 2-3:
The valves
of the heart
and how
they work.

From lower body

Right ventricle

Trunk and lower extremities

The coronary arteries

Three large coronary arteries and their many branches supply blood to the heart. As you can see in Figure 2-4, two coronary arteries branch off one main trunk, which is called the *left main coronary artery.* One of these branches runs down the front of the heart, so in medspeak, it is naturally called the *left anterior descending artery.* (*Anterior* is just a fancy word for front.) The second branch of the left main coronary artery circles around and supplies the side wall of the heart, so it is called the *left circumflex artery.* The third main coronary artery, which typically comes off of a separate trunk vessel, is called the *right coronary artery.* It supplies the back and bottom walls of the heart.

Significant narrowing of any of these coronary arteries causes angina, a symptom typically characterized as chest pain. (I discuss angina in detail in Chapter 4.) An acute, or sudden, blockage of one these arteries causes a heart attack, and, as a result, the heart muscle that formerly was supplied by the blocked artery dies.

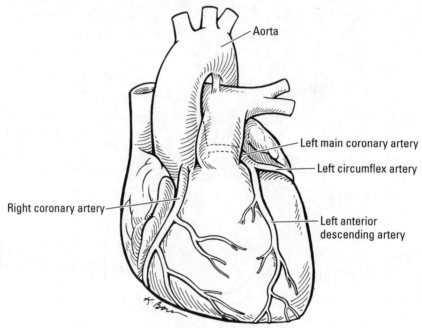

Aorta

Left main coronary artery

Left circumflex artery

Right coronary artery

Left anterior descending artery

K. Born

Figure 2-4:
The coronary arteries.

Mechanics tell you that the most important thing you can do to keep your car healthy is to change the oil frequently. Well, keeping your coronary arteries clear, free-flowing, and doing their job for the heart is the most important thing you can do to keep your heart healthy for a lifetime. Restoring blood flow to the heart and maintaining open arteries is the objective of a number of lifestyle, medical, and surgical treatments for coronary artery disease. This book shares a number of strategies you can use that your physician may prescribe to help you achieve this goal.

The electrical system

Would it surprise you to hear that the beating of your heart is controlled by an electrical system? Many folks are shocked (pun and double-entendre intended) to hear that's true. What's even more exciting is that your cardiac electric company is the mechanism that enables pacemakers and defibrillators (those dramatic standbys of TV doctor dramas — "Clear!") to work. This electrical system is controlled by a group of specialized cells that spontaneously discharge, sending electrical currents down specialized nerves and tissues, thus alerting all the other heart cells that it's time to discharge and causing the heart to contract, which for most folks is at a rate of about 70 to 80 times a minute when at rest. When any of these electrical structures becomes diseased or disordered, *arrhythmias* (ay-*rith*-mee-uhz), or heart rhythm disturbances, occur. (See Chapter 6 for more about arrhythmias.)

The pericardium

The entire heart is positioned in a thin sac called the *pericardium* (*peri* = around and *cardium* = heart; prounounced per-ry-*car*-dee-um). The thin-walled pericardium normally rests right up against the walls of the heart and is lubricated by a thin layer of body fluids that enable the heart to slide easily within it. However, this sac around the heart can become inflamed, resulting in chest discomfort or even compromised heart function. (You can check out these conditions, known as pericarditis, in Chapter 9).

Connecting Every Cell in Your Body: The Cardiovascular System

A pump is useless without the rest of the plumbing, which in your body is called the *cardiovascular system.* In the sections that follow, you can take a quick look at how it all fits together and functions.

The lungs

The lungs rest on either side of the heart and take up most of the space in the chest cavity, as shown in Figure 2-5. The lungs are composed of an intricate series of air sacs surrounded by a complex, highly branching network of blood vessels. Their sole purpose in life is to receive the deoxygenated blood from the heart, chock the red corpuscles full of fresh oxygen, and send them back to the heart for delivery to the body. This heart-to-lung-to-heart circuit functions as a low-pressure system to facilitate the rapid flow and reoxygenation of enormous amounts of blood. What that means is that the heart doesn't have to exert very great force with each contraction to move blood through this system.

A clot in a blood vessel in the lungs, otherwise known as a *pulmonary embolism,* and high blood pressure in the lungs' arteries, *pulmonary hypertension,* are two cardiac conditions related to the lungs. (For more about these conditions, see Chapter 9.)

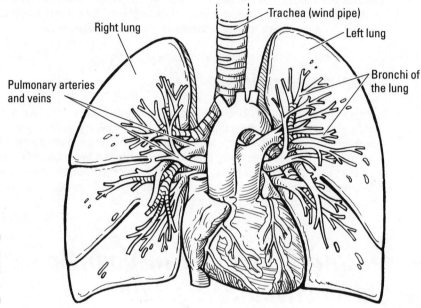

Right lung

Trachea (wind pipe)

Left lung

Bronchi of the lung

Pulmonary arteries and veins

Figure 2-5:
The heart
and lungs.

The arteries

As oxygenated blood returns to the left side of the heart, it is pumped out to the body through the *aorta,* the main artery of the body, and into the rest of the arterial system to feed the entire body with oxygenated blood. Because the body is fairly large compared to the size of the heart, the heart exerts enough force to push oxygenated blood throughout the body. However, arteries also have muscular walls that help push the blood along. The force exerted against resistance of the artery walls creates a high-pressure system that is very *elastic* to allow the arteries to expand or contract to meet the needs of various organs and muscles regardless of whether they're working or at rest.

So each time the left ventricle contracts, pumping blood into the arterial system, the arteries, in turn, expand to accept the surge of blood. However, this expansion of the arterial system doesn't occur as rapidly as the heart contracts. Therefore, when the heart relaxes, pressure still is in the arterial system and blood continues to move forward or out to the body. The contraction of the left ventricle is called *systole* (*sis*-tuh-lee). When the heart relaxes, the pressure falls somewhat as the blood continues to flow in the arterial system. This relaxation of the heart is called *diastole* (dye-*ass*-tuh-lee). Your *blood pressure* is measured by the amount of pressure in the arteries during the systole (contraction) and the diastole (relaxation). These measurements are represented by two numbers, one above the other. For example, one normal blood pressure reading is 110/70 mm Hg: The upper number is systolic pressure; the lower is diastolic pressure. High blood pressure, or *hypertension*, contributes to heart disease by stressing and damaging artery walls. (Read more about high blood pressure in Chapter 13.)

The capillaries

The arterial system divides and redivides into a system of ever smaller branches to distribute nourishing blood to each individual cell, ultimately ending up in a network of microscopic vessels called *capillaries,* which deliver oxygenated blood to the working cells of every organ and muscle in the body. This amazing network of branching microscopic vessels puts even the most complex digital network to shame! For example, a section of body tissue no bigger than the head of a pin has between 2,000 and 3,000 capillaries.

The veins

After oxygen leaves the capillary system, the deoxygenated blood and waste products from the cells are carried back through the body in the *veins.* The veins from the legs ultimately come together in a very large vein in the middle of the body called the *inferior vena cava* (*vee*-nuh *cay*-vuh), and all the veins in the upper part of the body come together in a large vein called the *superior vena cava.* These veins discharge blood into the right atrium of the heart to be pumped into the right ventricle and out to the lungs again to start the whole process over again. This circular flow of blood through the heart is illustrated earlier in Figure 2-3.

Keeping the Beat: How the Nervous System Controls Heart Rate

In addition to its internal electrical system, the heart has profound linkages to the nervous system that provide additional control of the heart rate. Two main branches of the involuntary nervous system interact with the heart — the sympathetic nervous system and the parasympathetic nervous system. In simple terms, the *sympathetic nervous system* helps the heart speed up, and the *parasympathetic nervous system* helps the heart slow down. I discuss rhythm problems in Chapter 6.

Sympathetic nervous system

The sympathetic nervous system typically directs the heart to speed up during periods of exercise or strong emotion. For example, you can feel your heart beat faster when you're angry, upset, or frightened. These responses probably go back to the survival needs of the earliest human history. Chapter 22 looks more fully at the reasons why. For now, however, I concentrate on the how. The sympathetic nervous system acts through direct nerve links to the heart and through chemical substances that reach the heart through the blood stream. In everyday speech, you can feel your adrenaline pumping.

When the heart speeds up, that quickened pace is known in medicine as *tacchycardia* (*tack*-ih-*car*-dee-uh). Of course, this is highly beneficial when you're exercising, but it is not so good when the accelerated rate results from disordered electrical impulses found in many people with heart disease. (See Chapter 6 for further discussion of heart rhythm problems.)

Parasympathetic nervous system

The parasympathetic branch of the nervous system acts as a trusty, unobtrusive housekeeper by keeping such functions as breathing and digestion perking along without any need for conscious thought on your part. Imagine how complex life would be if you had to stop and think each time you wanted to breathe. The parasympathetic nervous system can also direct the heart to slow down through direct nerve links to the heart and through release of a chemical called acetylcholine into the bloodstream.

The slowing of the heart is called *bradycardia* (*bray*-dee-*car*-dee-uh). When individuals are in great shape physically, they may have a healthy bradycardia. However, in certain diseased states, the heart rate can be too slow, resulting in inadequate blood flow to the tissues.

In certain circumstances, the parasympathetic nervous system can even be tricked into causing an inappropriately slow heart rate. The resulting brief period of inadequate blood flow to the brain usually causes a fainting episode. Fainting is the brain's safety valve because when it decides the heart is not sending it enough blood, the brain sends the body crashing to the ground, where in a horizontal position, the brain automatically gets its share of the blood flow, regardless of whether the heart is going fast or slow.

Inviting Heart Disease: The Couch Potato Connection

Now that you know what all the parts of the cardiovascular system are, I can show you how they work together and how easy starting down the slippery slope that leads toward heart disease can be. You can start with the favorite position of most Americans — relaxing on the couch.

The view from the couch

While you're sitting still, your heart is beating at 70 to 80 contractions per minute (unless you're very fit, but more about that later). With each contraction, the right ventricle discharges about three-quarters of the blood it contains into the vessels of the lungs where it receives oxygen. At the same time, the left ventricle is discharging about three-quarters of the blood that it contains into the aorta and arterial system to feed the oxygen to all the organs and muscles. All four heart valves work together to control blood flow into and out of the heart, making sure that no blood flows in the wrong direction. Wouldn't it be nice if traffic systems were so efficient!

The arterial system dilates, or expands, each time the left ventricle empties into it and speeds blood on its way to the various working tissues. How much blood goes to each tissue is determined by what that particular muscle or organ needs to do. When you eat a big meal, for example, the heart, brain, parasympathetic nervous system, and arteries all decide that more blood needs to go to the organs in the gastrointestinal tract to help them with the work of digesting that low-fat, cardiac-healthy meal you just ate.

The view from the track

Say that after reading this book and consulting with your physician, you decide that you're going to exercise regularly. (Good idea!) Exercise poses a different challenge to the heart compared to rest. Extra blood flow must go to muscles used in exercising and to the coronary arteries that feed the heart muscle itself so that it can pump out the extra blood required during your exercise exertion.

Fortunately, this extra work is no problem for a healthy heart. Once again, all systems work in concert. Extra blood is pumped from the heart, and extra blood flows down the coronary arteries, which dilate to accept this extra flow. The heart valves continue to direct the blood in the proper direction, and the electrical system, with a little boost from the nervous system, starts generating more beats per minute. At the same time, the cardiac muscle relaxes a little bit, enabling more blood to be pumped out during each beat.

In addition, the nervous system, in conjunction with the arterial system, causes

- Some parts of the arterial circulation to expand or dilate, sending more blood to the working muscles that need it
- Other parts to constrict or narrow, diverting blood away from areas where it is not as active during exertion

The good news is that if you exert yourself on a regular basis, your heart and the rest of your cardiovascular system begin to become more efficient and prepare for the regular exercise sessions. That's true even if you've been diagnosed with heart disease or had a heart attack or other heart event. For that reason, physicians prescribe specific types of carefully monitored activities and exercises as part of treatment and rehabilitation programs for heart disease.

Sliding down the Slippery Slope toward Heart Disease

When all parts of the heart and cardiovascular system are healthy and functioning well together, it is a beautiful system. But the heart is a muscle. And like any muscle, it works best when you keep it in shape and avoid injury.

The conditioned heart

A conditioned heart is stronger and better able to meet the demands the body places on it. Human bodies were designed to be in motion. And the motion of physical activity keeps the heart well tuned, the benefits of which are numerous:

✔ Literally hundreds of studies have shown that individuals who adopt the simple habit of daily physical activity substantially reduce their risk of developing various heart problems, most notably coronary artery disease.

✔ The conditioned heart enables individuals to accomplish the activities of daily living with comfort and without running out of breath and energy.

✔ The more conditioned the heart, the lower the resting heart rate, and the less work the heart has to do in a lifetime.

✔ Studies also show that, with appropriate activity, hearts damaged by disease or injury can regain conditioning that enhances health and function and may even contribute to the reversal of some aspects of disease.

The deconditioned heart

In contrast to the active individual, the individual who leads a sedentary lifestyle can actually experience a deconditioned heart. The deconditioned heart is less efficient at doing its work and has to work harder to get adequate blood flow throughout the body. You're a prime candidate for a deconditioned heart if you answer "yes" to these questions or others like them:

✔ Do you avoid the stairs because climbing two or three flights leaves you extremely short of breath?

✔ Do you circle a parking lot numerous times looking for a space right in front of the store to make sure that you don't have to walk much?

✔ Do you watch sports on television rather than participate in them with friends and family?

✔ On a nice day, do you pop a DVD into the player rather than take a walk?

For many people a deconditioned heart is the first step in a slow slide down the long slope toward a sick heart.

The diseased heart

A sedentary lifestyle coupled with unhealthy practices such as poor nutrition, weight gain, cigarette smoking, or certain other health conditions, such as high blood pressure, high cholesterol, or diabetes, can severely alter the basic cardiac structures and lead to a disordered anatomy that can create a very unhappy destiny. A short list of the things that can go wrong includes blocked arteries, high cholesterol, high blood pressure, angina, heart attack, heart failure, and sudden death. The bottom line: Many of the cardiac problems that people experience are brought on by years of neglect and failure to abide by even the most basic of cardiac-healthy lifestyle principles. (Nature makes a few mistakes, too, but even in those cases, personal choices often complicate the problem.)

The good news is that even if you've been diagnosed as at risk for heart disease or as having it, and even if you've experienced specific heart problems, paying attention to the basic principles of a cardiac-healthy lifestyle in conjunction with the medications and procedures of your treatment plan can help you turn things around.

Chapter 3

Recognizing Your Risk of Coronary Heart Disease

- -

In This Chapter

▶ Defining risk factors for heart disease

▶ Identifying the big six risk factors that you can control

▶ Watching for three risk factors you cannot control

▶ Staying alert for emerging risk factors

- -

*I*n the history of medicine, risk factors are a relatively new concept. In fact, before World War II, when men (and it usually was men) and women died suddenly, it was thought to be an act of God. Even when people knew that someone died of a heart attack, the cause of the heart attack wasn't linked to any personal habits or actions. How else can you explain sending soldiers off to battle with cigarettes as a reward for a job well done, advertising Camel cigarettes as "the doctor's choice," or not thinking twice about consuming enormous steaks without trimming the fat? Borrowing a phrase that unfortunately was co-opted by a cigarette manufacturer, "You've come a long way, baby!"

Heart disease takes many forms (see Part II of this book for more about them), and established and emerging risk factors contribute to each form of heart disease in complex ways. In this chapter, I discuss the risk factors for the most common form, coronary artery disease (CAD) or *atherosclerosis*. Paying close attention to the roles the various risk factors play and remembering that most of them can be controlled can go a long way toward slowing or even reversing CAD.

Defining Risk Factors

What is a risk factor anyway? Just as the name suggests, a *risk factor* is something that increases your chances of developing a chronic condition — that is, an ongoing health condition that you must live with. In the case of cardiac health, a risk factor is a personal habit, practice, or physical characteristic or condition that increases the likelihood that you'll develop CAD. In other words, risk factors contribute to the progression of the disease or condition.

Doctors continually are discovering more and more about the risk factors for CAD, primarily through a number of long-term studies of very large groups of people, including the Framingham Heart Study, which has followed the lifestyles and health records of 10,000 men and women in great detail for more than 50 years.

Risk factors for heart disease are classified as either *major risk factors,* which at least double your risk of heart disease, or *other risk factors,* which do not, according to the current research data, demonstrate a level of danger on par with that of the major risk factors. Nevertheless, other risk factors can contribute to your chances of getting heart disease in significant ways. Being male (sorry, guys) and experiencing stress are other risk factors. Major risk factors include:

- ✔ Cigarette smoking
- ✔ Diabetes
- ✔ Elevated cholesterol and low HDL
- ✔ Family history of premature heart disease
- ✔ Hypertension
- ✔ Inactive lifestyle
- ✔ Increasing age
- ✔ Obesity

Chasing down some new leads

Every day scientists are finding out and publishing more about other risk factors that contribute to CAD. For example, newer studies have added to the knowledge of suspected risk factors, such as a high consumption of alcohol, elevated levels of homocysteine (an amino acid), low levels of antioxidants, and abnormal blood clotting. As continuing research provides more data, many of these conditions or markers will be confirmed and classified as either major or other risk factors.

Checking out promising new research

In thousands of research laboratories and institutions around the world, ongoing research explores potential causes and risks for heart disease. One area of particular interest is the exploration of complex genetic links to heart disease. During the last few years, the mapping of all the genes in the human body, the human genome, has opened promising avenues of research into possible genetic causes for complex cardiovascular traits. Scientists and physicians have only begun tapping into the potential that genomic medical research may hold for treatment and even prevention of various heart conditions.

Multiplying risks — double trouble and more

One aspect of risk factors that makes them particularly dangerous is that their effects multiply, rather than merely add up, whenever you exhibit two or more of them. As you can see in Figure 3-1, which is based on data from the Framingham Heart Study, individuals with only a single risk factor actually double their chances of developing heart disease. When two risk factors are present, the possibility quadruples. And, worse yet, when three risk factors join forces, the possibility of your developing heart disease increases 8 to 20 times! If you think that's bad news, listen to this: Having two and three risk factors is not unusual. In fact, risk factors have a distinct tendency to occur in clusters (see the section "Being obese or overweight" later in this chapter).

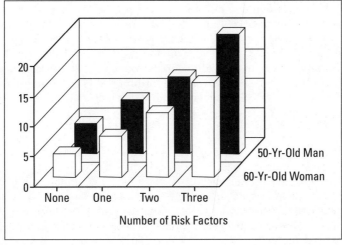

Figure 3-1: Eight-year risk of developing CHD (CAD) per 1,000, according to number of coronary risk factors.

Framingham Heart Study

Heading off trouble by controlling risk

For most risk factors, what you helped create, you can also change through:

- **Primary prevention:** By controlling risk factors before the onslaught of CAD, you can substantially lower your chances of ever developing coronary heart disease by

  - Lowering your blood pressure

  - Lowering your cholesterol

  - Quitting smoking

  - Becoming more active (exercising)

  - Losing weight

- **Secondary prevention:** If you already have CAD, attempting to bring these same factors under control usually decreases your risk of having further complications and manifestations from CAD.

Controlling or treating a particular risk factor may mean different things for different individuals. One size does not fit all. For example, a young woman with a mildly elevated cholesterol level — say 215 mg/dl — but no other risk factors may require only some healthful modifications in diet and physical activity. On the other hand, a 60-year-old man who's already suffered a heart attack and has the same level of elevated cholesterol may require immediate, aggressive treatment to lower his cholesterol levels. (See Chapter 14 for more about cholesterol.)

Because a young woman with an elevated cholesterol level has a relatively greater risk of developing coronary heart disease than a young woman who doesn't have an elevated cholesterol level, she needs to work with her physician on modifying lifestyle habits to lower her cholesterol. Her situation is not as immediately threatening and therefore doesn't need to be treated as aggressively as that of the 60-year-old man with heart disease and elevated cholesterol. Because his elevated cholesterol comes in the context of his already having heart disease, therapy for him needs to be much more intensive. In treating heart disease, controlling risk factors is an important part of every treatment regimen.

Identifying Six Risk Factors That You Can Control

Although risk factors often are classified as *major* factors or *other* factors, dividing them into the ones you *can* modify and the ones you *cannot* modify probably is more enlightening. So that's the way I discuss them, starting with the risk factors that you can tackle successfully.

Having hypertension — high blood pressure

Landmark studies conducted in the 1960s put to rest any serious doubt that elevated blood pressure, or *hypertension,* represents a substantial risk for developing CAD and stroke. Hypertension appears to be particularly dangerous in terms of the likelihood of developing a stroke. (For an in-depth discussion of hypertension, see Chapter 13. For more about stroke, see Chapter 8.)

Hypertension is extremely common in the United States, probably because of the nutritional habits, propensity to gain weight, and sedentary lifestyle of most Americans. More than one-fourth of the entire adult population in the United States suffers from hypertension. By the time an individual reaches age 60, he or she has a greater than 60 percent chance of having elevated blood pressure. More than 31 percent of people with high blood pressure don't know they have it — no wonder it's called the "silent killer."

Once again, the good news is that daily habits and practices, such as appropriate weight control, sound nutrition, and regular physical activity can profoundly diminish the likelihood of your ever developing hypertension in the first place and can significantly contribute to the effective treatment of elevated blood pressure. (For more about these healthful practices, see Chapters 20 and 21.) In fact, controlling blood pressure within normal levels is an important part of both primary and secondary prevention of heart disease (and kidney disease, the other great health risk of hypertension).

Having elevated cholesterol

By now, almost everyone knows having a high cholesterol level in your blood is a bad thing. When it comes to being at risk of developing CAD, however, an elevated level of blood cholesterol is one of a number of *lipid problems* (problems with fats in the blood) that significantly elevate your risk of heart disease. The abnormalities that are particularly dangerous include elevated total cholesterol, elevated LDL cholesterol, low HDL cholesterol, elevated triglycerides, or any combination of the four.

The good news is that by following appropriate lifestyle measures and, in some instances, using effective medicines that now are available, this risk factor for CAD can be effectively managed. You can get all the definitions, evidence, and strategies for better controlling cholesterol levels in Chapter 14.

Using tobacco

With all the information available about health, heart disease, and cigarette smoking, smokers who fail to understand that smoking poses a very serious threat to their health must have been hiding incommunicado in a wilderness cave for the last 40 years. Reams of data present a very stark, negative picture: Cigarette smoking (and the use of other tobacco products) is the leading cause of premature death in the United States each year, claiming more than 400,000 lives.

Although cigarette smoking has declined, unfortunately about 26 percent of adult men and 22 percent of adult women still smoke cigarettes. Shockingly, although many adults successfully struggle to quit cigarette smoking, an estimated 3,000 children start smoking every day.

The health consequences of cigarette smoking are severe. Smoking

- ✔ Triples the risk of developing heart disease and increases the risk of developing lung cancer by a whopping 3,000 percent.
- ✔ Increases the risk of harming the health of others. Individuals with CAD can have angina attacks provoked merely by being in a smoke-filled room.
- ✔ Tends to lower HDL cholesterol (the good guys).

In an otherwise bleak picture, the outstanding good news is that stopping smoking

> ✔ Lowers the risk of developing CAD and significantly improves the health outlook for individuals who have heart disease.
>
> ✔ Can add two to three years to your life expectancy.
>
> ✔ Improves blood lipids. In one study, LDL cholesterol decreased more than 5 percent and HDL cholesterol increased more than 3 percent in individuals who stopped cigarette smoking.

Quitting is so important (and so tough) that Chapter 23 is devoted to the facts and strategies you need so that you can find the ways and means — and support — to stamp out smoking in your life.

Being physically inactive

In 1994, faced with overwhelming evidence, the American Heart Association added the first new major factor in 25 years — a physically inactive lifestyle — to the list of risks for developing CAD. Physical inactivity is defined as a major factor, in part, because it also contributes significantly to a number of the other major risk factors, such as high blood pressure, perhaps elevated blood cholesterol, and often obesity. But if you get off your duff and get active, you can turn this sad picture around. (See Chapter 21 for help.) A physically active lifestyle not only reduces the specific risk that inactivity poses for heart disease, it also helps lessen or eradicate several of the other major risk factors for heart disease.

Being obese or overweight

In 1998, obesity joined the list of major independent risk factors for developing CAD. Like physical inactivity, obesity also contributes to many other risk factors, including hypertension and elevated cholesterol, and other abnormal lipid levels.

Unfortunately, during the last ten years, the prevalence of obesity has grown a shocking 66 percent, according to the Centers for Disease Control. More than one in every three adults is now considered obese. By *obese,* I mean weighing at least 20 percent more than desirable body weight. That's not as fat as most people think, either. For example, if your optimal weight is 150 pounds and you weigh 180 — just 30 pounds overweight — you are technically obese even if you think you still look pretty good. Nearly two-thirds of adults are overweight.

Being obese increases the risk of CAD in a number of different ways that include:

✔ Interacting negatively with many other risk factors for developing CAD, such as high blood pressure, Type 2 diabetes, and cholesterol problems.

✔ Clustering of risk factors. Obese people are particularly susceptible to a clustering of risk factors. In fact, an obese individual is

   • 70 percent more likely to be affected by at least one other risk factor for heart disease.

   • 50 percent more likely to be affected by at least two other risk factors for heart disease.

   • 20 percent to 25 percent more likely to be affected by three other risk factors for heart disease!

✔ Serving as a forerunner to dangerous lipid abnormalities that increase the risk of heart disease, including:

   • Elevated blood triglycerides.

   • Elevated LDL cholesterol levels.

   • Depressed HDL cholesterol levels.

Carrying extra weight around the abdomen (sometimes called *abdominal obesity* or *apple-shaped obesity*) is particularly dangerous in terms of its risk of coronary heart disease.

Overweight individuals, who, in addition to excess weight, often face one or more other risk factors for CAD, are particularly susceptible to dying from heart disease because of probable abnormalities caused by fat cells in general and abdominal fat cells in particular.

If you're overweight, regardless of whether you have heart disease, you need to make a point of talking to your doctor about whether you show signs of having other risk factors for heart disease in addition to obesity. The odds are that you do.

If you've been diagnosed with heart disease and are overweight, then be sure to discuss these issues with your physician. Weight loss in and of itself is a highly effective way of reducing multiple risk factors for heart disease. In Chapters 20 and 21, I discuss the principles and techniques of nutrition and effective weight management and of developing an activity program that can help you create a lifestyle plan to achieve these goals.

Remember, obese people do not die because they are too fat; they die of heart disease.

Having diabetes mellitus

Approximately 17 million people in the United States, or 6.2 percent of the population, suffer from diabetes mellitus. About 90 percent to 95 percent of these individuals have Type 2 or adult onset diabetes. Diabetes represents a significant risk factor for coronary heart disease. In fact, coronary heart disease is by far the leading cause of death in individuals with diabetes.

Individuals with diabetes often have multiple blood lipid abnormalities including elevated blood triglycerides and elevated LDL cholesterol and a depressed HDL cholesterol. Having this particular constellation of lipid abnormalities spells triple trouble! For reasons that to date are not totally clear, women with diabetes have an even greater risk of developing heart disease than men with diabetes.

Recent compelling research also indicates that individuals who have some degree of insulin resistance or glucose intolerance — test results that put them in the "prediabetic" category — also have elevated risk of heart disease.

By working with your physician if you have diabetes, however, you can lower many of the complications of diabetes and also control your blood lipids. Daily steps that you can take to help you control diabetes include weight loss if you're overweight, regular physical activity, and proper nutritional habits.

Watching for Risk Factors That You Cannot Modify

Now I come to three risk factors that you can't modify: your age, gender, and family history (see the list that follows). Having one or more of these nonmodifiable risk factors makes it particularly important that you pay close attention to the risk factors that you *can* modify.

- ✔ **Age:** Age is considered a significant risk factor for CAD for men who are older than 45 and for women who are older than 55 or have undergone premature menopause.

- ✔ **Gender:** Men are more likely to develop CAD than women. Furthermore, the onset of symptoms of CAD typically occurs ten years later in women than in men; however, pointing out that CAD remains the number-one killer in *both* men and women in the United States is important. CAD becomes particularly prevalent in women after menopause. After age 65, men and women have approximately the same risk for developing CAD.

✔ **Family history:** CAD tends to occur more frequently in some families than in others. Coming from a family in which premature coronary heart disease has occurred clearly increases your risk of developing CAD. By *premature coronary heart disease* I mean a diagnosed heart attack or a sudden death before age 55 in males or age 65 in females. Having a first-degree relative (father, mother, brother, or sister) who fits this description qualifies as a risk factor.

Paying Attention to Emerging Risk Factors

Research continues to identify factors that may increase or decrease your risk for developing CAD. Although conclusive verification isn't yet available, discussing the following potential risk factors with your physician still is a worthwhile proposition:

✔ **Stress and Type A personality:** Without a doubt, physical and emotional linkages exist between the mind and the heart. Research evidence increasingly suggests that an individual's response to acute and chronic stress from various environmental pressures and psychosocial factors, such as isolation, anger, and depression, may contribute to heart disease. For example, individuals who exhibit Type A behaviors — people who persistently are rushed and unhappy and particularly those who face the world with high levels of hostility — are at increased risk for developing CAD. Many promising areas of research into the effects of stress on heart disease remain. The potential risks of stress and benefits of properly addressing it are clear enough, and if you experience high levels of stress in your life exploring ways of lowering it is worthwhile. (See Chapter 22 for strategies.)

✔ **Alcohol:** The relationship between alcohol and CAD is complex. Several studies show that moderate alcohol consumption may actually be associated with decreased risk of CAD. *Moderate consumption* means no more than one to two glasses of wine per day, one to two beers per day, or one and a half ounces of distilled spirits a day. Individuals who do not currently consume alcohol, however, should not use these findings as a justification to start. Furthermore, higher levels of alcohol consumption — three alcoholic drinks per day or more — are associated with an increased risk of high blood pressure and CAD (and motor vehicle accidents, for that matter), so stick with moderation.

✔ **Homocysteine:** *Homocysteine* is an amino acid that serves as a building block of proteins in the body. However, some studies show that elevated concentrations of homocysteine in the blood can be associated with increased risk of CAD. Fortunately, relatively simple measures, in particular taking additional *folic acid* (also referred to as *folate*) can reduce elevated levels of homocysteine.

Most scientists encourage people who need to restrict blood levels of homocysteine to consume 400 micrograms of folate per day. Because this information is new, you need to consult with your physician about whether your blood homocysteine level needs to be checked. Although daily consumption of 400 mcg of folic acid may be a reasonable health decision where the risk of developing CAD is concerned, it is absolutely mandatory for women of childbearing age, because it helps prevent birth defects related to brain and spine development, including spina bifida.

✔ **Low levels of antioxidants:** In recent years, antioxidants have been hyped by the popular media as the cure *du jour* for several conditions including risk of heart disease. Several studies have supported the concept that low levels of antioxidants in blood may increase the risk of developing CAD. These findings have led some physicians to recommend that individuals who are either at increased risk for coronary heart disease or who have established heart disease take supplementary antioxidants such as vitamin E, vitamin C, and/or beta-carotene. This recommendation, which remains controversial, isn't included as part of the current generally accepted recommendations for reducing standard risk factors. But further studies are underway to clarify whether supplementing antioxidants is a reasonable recommendation. More recent studies in this area suggest that antioxidants don't lower the risk of heart disease.

✔ **Abnormal blood clotting:** During the last ten years, substantial evidence has emerged indicating that how your blood clots is part of the process of acute CAD. Certain rare clotting abnormalities clearly increase the risk of coronary heart disease for some individuals. But at this time, using blood-clotting parameters to determine an individual's risk of developing CAD is highly experimental. If you have questions about whether this rare problem relates to you, discuss it with your physician.

✔ **Markers or factors for specific heart conditions:** Beyond continuing research on the contribution of major risk factors to heart disease, some of the most promising current research concerns identifying specific *markers,* or factors that may indicate an increased risk of developing a specific condition or event. In addition to discovering how such markers work physically, researchers are exploring the potential clinical use of such markers to help diagnose and treat patients. The following examples give you an idea of the nature and promise of such research.

- **Elevated C-Reactive Protein:** Elevated blood levels of *C-Reactive Protein (CRP),* a marker that increases during systemic inflammation (inflammation that affects the whole body), are associated with increased heart attacks and other heart events caused by blood clots. Studies consistently show that higher levels of CRP predict a higher risk of heart attack.

  High CRP is particularly associated with the increased occurrence of new heart events and a lower survival rate in individuals who have unstable angina or have had a heart attack. CRP may also prove useful in predicting a higher risk of heart attack for healthy individuals who don't have elevated cholesterol or CAD symptoms.

  In addition to broadening the populations studied beyond men and women of European heritage, ongoing research continues to explore ways in which CRP levels may provide indicators that are useful in preventing, diagnosing, and treating various manifestations of cardiovascular disease.

- **Lp(a) cholesterol:** This genetic variation of LDL cholesterol (the bad guys) is clearly associated with a greater risk of prematurely developing CAD. Research into how this marker may be useful diagnostically is one aspect of ongoing research.

- **Factor V Leiden:** About 2 percent to 7 percent of persons of European descent have this variation of the factor V gene, a variant that promotes the formation of blood clots in blood vessels. Persons with V Leiden are at greater risk of developing heart attack, stroke, and deep vein thrombosis. But risk among individuals with this variant appears to vary widely. Current research into gene modifiers is exploring ways to accurately identify individuals who are at greatest risk.

Part II
Identifying the Many Forms of Heart Disease

The 5th Wave   By Rich Tennant

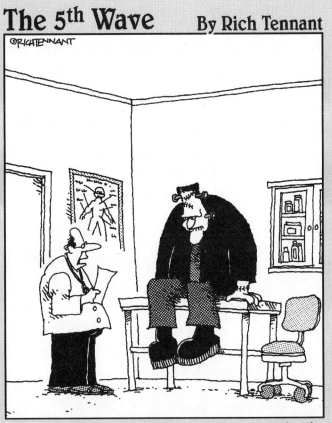

"It's important that you get your high blood pressure under control. It could not only affect your kidneys and heart, but also your current brain."

In this part . . .

Get the basic information you need to help you understand coronary heart disease and its manifestations, including angina and heart attack. I also provide an overview of the many strategies and techniques that modern science and medicine offer to diagnose and treat these conditions. I then take the same approach to understanding other important forms of heart disease, including heart rhythm problems, heart failure (congestive heart failure), stroke, and other less common conditions.

Chapter 4

Understanding the Onset of Coronary Artery Disease, Angina, and Unstable Angina

*N*early 13 million people alive today in the United States suffer from some form of coronary artery disease (CAD). Every 29 seconds, an American suffers a complication of CAD; every minute, another dies from it. CAD is the most significant chronic condition and the leading cause of death for all segments of society.

But Americans have been fighting back. During the last decade, the death rate from CAD has declined more than 25 percent. This number can decline even further when you understand how CAD develops and what you can do to prevent and to control it to get the most out of life.

If you or someone you love is diagnosed with CAD or if you simply want to work on prevention, empowerment starts with discovering the facts about how CAD begins and progresses.

In this chapter, I discuss first the silent precursors and early stages that have no symptoms and then look at *angina* and *unstable angina,* two types of chest pain that often first manifest heart disease for many people. In Chapter 5, I discuss heart attacks, and in Chapter 6, I talk about arrhythmia, heart rhythm problems — the acute problems that represent the next steps in the progression of CAD.

Defining CAD, or Atherosclerosis

Coronary artery disease (also known as CAD, *coronary heart disease — CHD, coronary atherosclerosis,* or *coronary arteriosclerosis*) is the slow, progressive narrowing of the three main arteries (and their branches) that supply blood to the heart. This narrowing of the arteries gradually starves the heart muscle of the high level of oxygenated blood that it needs to function properly. A lack of adequate blood supply to the heart typically produces symptoms that range from angina and unstable angina (see "Defining Angina" and "Defining Unstable Angina" later in this chapter) to heart attack or sudden death.

Narrowing arteries that are characteristic of CAD result from the gradual buildup of fatty deposits called *plaque,* or *lesions,* on their interior walls. *Atherosclerosis,* the most common medical term for CAD, comes from two Greek words — *athero* (paste, gruel) and *sclerosis* (hardness) — that may give you a graphic image of hardened sludge. Not a pretty picture, is it? But it's an apt image for these deposits of cholesterol, other fats, cellular wastes, platelets, calcium, and other substances. These deposits typically start with fatty streaks and grow to large bumps that distort the artery and block its interior where the blood must flow. Some plaques are stable and others are unstable or vulnerable to cracking or rupturing, which often leads to an artery-blocking blood clot and subsequent heart attack. I discuss the whole process in the next section.

The disease process that leads to advanced atherosclerosis starts with small changes in the artery wall and takes years to develop to a point where the narrowing arteries may produce symptoms or negatively affect your health. The sections that follow profile that development process.

During the last 15 to 20 years, evidence from extensive population studies and clinical research has increased doctors' understanding of the many factors and pathways that contribute to the beginnings and progress of CAD. The next section provides an overview that shares medical science's best understanding right now; however, you need to remember that new studies continually add to the knowledge of this complex, multifaceted disease.

Discovering what causes CAD

Biomedical evidence suggests that at least three major factors (combined with numerous lesser ones) probably play a primary role in triggering and fostering the disease process of atherosclerosis:

✔ **Chronic injury to the endothelium:** Damage to the *endothelium,* or lining of the artery walls, is largely the result of the action of such risk factors as high blood pressure (Chapter 13), smoking (Chapter 23), elevated levels of cholesterol and other lipids (fats) in the blood (Chapter 14), and diabetes. The damage

   • Gives cholesterol and other cells that eventually form plaques a way to attach to the endothelial lining or enter the artery walls.

   • Appears to cause inflammation and activate the cellular repair team of the immune system, which speeds to injury sites.

✔ **Elevated cholesterol and other lipids in the blood:** When blood levels of cholesterol, particularly LDL (low density lipoprotein) cholesterol, are too high, excess LDL cholesterol is deposited on the endothelial lining of arteries where special receptor cells latch on to the LDL molecules. This trapped LDL can damage the cells by a process called oxidation. The oxidation attracts certain protective cells already in artery walls and circulating in the blood that engulf the oxidized excess lipid. Soon other protective mechanisms such as platelets, T-cells, and growth factors for smooth muscle cells are working hard to restore the damage from excess lipid. Unfortunately, this biological process, which is intended to restore the artery wall to normal, overdoes it. As the process seals off the excess lipids, it actually creates cholesterol-rich pockets covered with scar tissue. These lesions narrow the arteries and typically deform artery walls as they grow larger.

✔ **Inflammation:** From its earliest stages atherosclerosis appears to trigger inflammation, the body's first line of defense against injury and infection. Evidence to date suggests that inflammation serves as a mediator in the disease progression by recruiting various immune system repair and fighter cells. The exact pathways by which inflammation exerts its influence remain unclear, but scientists are researching a number of inflammation markers that may help physicians diagnose and treat persons at high risk of CAD in its early stages when lifestyle and medical therapies may halt or even reverse the disease. Such markers may prove particularly useful for at-risk individuals who have few or no risk factors (see Chapter 3).

Progressing from fatty streaks to large plaques

Biological factors that contribute to the development of CAD are present from birth and perform vital functions that enable the human body to grow and resist infection. As a consequence, all human beings are born with the potential to develop CAD. In fact, the first visible signs of CAD, fatty streaks on inner artery walls, frequently occur in children, teens, and young adults. Decades and the presence of various risk factors are required for the streaks to develop into intermediate (moderate-sized, symptomless) and advanced (larger, symptom-producing) plaques. Figure 4-1 illustrates the typical but gradual development and progression of CAD.

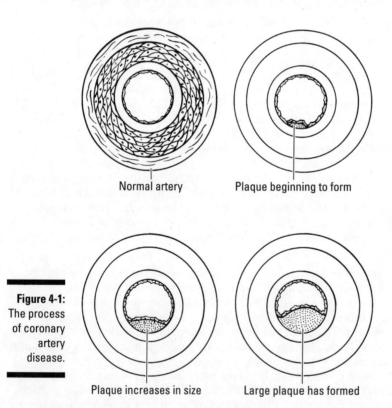

Normal artery   Plaque beginning to form

Figure 4-1:
The process
of coronary
artery
disease.

Plaque increases in size   Large plaque has formed

Starting with fatty streaks

As you can see from the upper-left image in Figure 4-1, a healthy artery has several layers:

- ✔ A protective outer sheath
- ✔ A layer of active muscular cells in the middle that enables the artery to contract
- ✔ An inner layer of smooth muscle cells, called the *intima,* that has a one-cell-deep lining, the endothelium

Changes that lead to atherosclerosis begin with the endothelium and intima.

As a basic building block for every cell, cholesterol constantly circulates in the blood along with other substances that are vital for life. Besides cholesterol, the immune system also is on guard in the normal cardiovascular system. Protective cells and substances, such as platelets and white cells, circulate in the blood. In fact, isolated protective cells known as *macrophages* hang out in the healthy artery lining.

However, when LDL cholesterol attaches to the artery lining, macrophages engulf it. When excess LDL is present on the artery lining, more fighter cells (known as *monocytes*) circulating in the blood enter the lining and transform into macrophages.

As these macrophages engulf the cholesterol, they transform into *macrophage foam cells,* which usually appear as yellow fatty streaks visible on the interior artery walls. When the cholesterol level is controlled and plenty of HDL cholesterol (the good guys) is present to carry away LDL, then these fatty streaks can be halted or reversed. (For the complete story about cholesterol and controlling it, see Chapter 14.) But when excess cholesterol and/or other risk factors are present, the deposits may continue growing, gradually becoming larger lesions that are more complexly involved in the artery walls.

Growing to moderate, intermediate types of plaque

In the presence of normal mechanical forces, such as the impact of flowing blood against artery walls and risk factors that can injure artery walls, many fatty streaks begin growing into larger deposits. More cholesterol and other lipid (fat) particles migrate into the artery walls. This happens particularly in areas where the intima has thickened, probably to adapt to mechanical forces exerted on the arteries. More and more fatty substances aren't taken into macrophages or the smooth muscle cells, but rather they begin pooling between them. At that point, a thin layer of intimal tissue begins forming a cap to contain this lipid pool. Other substances such as cytokines and growth factors may also play a role in forming the cap and helping it continue to grow. The formation and growth of the cap mark the transition from *intermediate* lesions to what medspeak terms *advanced* (and typically more dangerous) *lesions.*

Becoming advanced atherosclerotic plaques

As plaques continue to grow, they reach a condition and size that may produce symptoms such as angina, unstable angina, or even heart attack or stroke. The various advanced types of *atherosclerotic plaques* are characterized by a well-defined lipid core that is contained by a cap composed of layers of smooth muscle cells and other substances.

At first this cap appears to be nearly normal intimal layers. But as the plaque grows larger, the composition of the cap's layers changes, becoming more fibrous, or scarlike, as substances such as collagen and calcium enter the mix.

Some advanced plaques are stable, but others are vulnerable to cracking or rupture. When a crack or tear occurs, the lipid core is exposed to arterial blood from which sticky platelets may trigger the formation of a blood clot intended to repair the break. The clot, however, enlarges the size of the plaque. Some plaques grow larger by a cyclical process of cracking and clotting, which gradually narrows the artery. The plaques that are more vulnerable to cracking are more likely to form a clot that totally blocks the artery and causes a sudden event such as a heart attack or stroke. So looking briefly at the difference between plaques is important.

Differentiating between stable and unstable plaques

As individual plaques grow to moderate size and begin exhibiting the rich lipid core and thin fibrous cap associated with the first level of advanced lesions, they appear to be more vulnerable to rupture and dangerous clot formation than larger, older, thicker plaques. Bigger doesn't necessarily mean more vulnerable, either. The most vulnerable plaques, which can give rise to the deadliest heart attacks, typically block the vessel by only about 40 percent to 50 percent.

Medical scientists and physicians are particularly interested in ways to accurately identify these types of vulnerable plaques, because they seem to be responsible for the majority of sudden acute cardiovascular events, including heart attack, cardiac arrest, and stroke. Figure 4-2 illustrates the way in which such a process suddenly blocks an artery and causes an acute event.

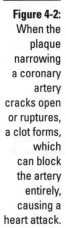

Figure 4-2:
When the plaque narrowing a coronary artery cracks open or ruptures, a clot forms, which can block the artery entirely, causing a heart attack.

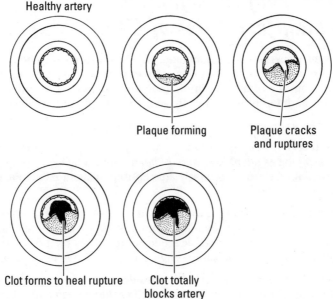

Healthy artery

Plaque forming

Plaque cracks and ruptures

Clot forms to heal rupture

Clot totally blocks artery

Current evidence suggests that stable plaques typically have thicker, more fibrous caps with few inflammatory cells and more calcification, which make the cap tougher. Stable plaques also appear to have fewer lipids within. Although stable plaques often are large, the edges or shoulders of the lesion usually are smooth and tapered.

Unstable plaques, by contrast, are smaller in size but are very rich in cholesterol and incorporate many more inflammatory cells, which release chemicals that degrade the fibrous cap. Unstable plaques often appear structurally weak. In addition, the thinner cap may be easily ruptured or torn by a number of forces, ranging from the normal flow of blood at high stress points in the arterial system to sudden pressures such as suddenly increased blood pressure from exertion.

Tests and techniques that accurately identify and assess unstable plaque would enhance the ability of physicians to identify individuals who may be at greater risk of acute events and set up measures for primary and secondary prevention.

Recognizing the symptoms and manifestations of CAD

Because every person is an individual, physical responses to progressive coronary artery disease vary. Not every individual with CAD has every manifestation and symptom of the condition. Individuals likewise experience specific symptoms in different ways. But these manifestations are typical:

- **Nothing:** Many people can have significant CAD but experience no discomfort or other sign of the disease. That's why this condition is known in medicine as *silent ischemia. Ischemia* means lack of blood flow. People with diabetes are particularly susceptible to silent ischemia, but others can have it, too.

- **Angina:** More formally known as *angina pectoris,* angina is typified by temporary chest pain, usually during exertion. This pain usually is felt as a tightness or uncomfortable feeling across the chest or up to the neck and jaw, not as a sharp stab. Angina also may have other manifestations.

- **Unstable angina:** Chest pain that is new, occurs when you're at rest, or suddenly grows more severe is called *unstable angina.* It's a medical emergency.

- **Heart attack:** Completely cutting off blood flow to a coronary artery causes an acute heart attack, or *myocardial infarction (MI),* the most severe result of CAD. The closure can be gradual or the result of a blood clot. (See also Chapter 5.)

- **Sudden death:** The cause of sudden death from CAD often is a rhythm problem such as ventricular tachycardia or ventricular fibrillation (see Chapter 6). These rhythm problems sometimes occur in the setting of an acute heart attack. I've highlighted it here to make the point that the first indication or symptom for many people that they have CAD is a fatal cardiac arrest or heart attack. How many people? It's hard to say exactly, but 250,000 sudden cardiac deaths occur each year, and the American Heart Association indicates that about half of all deaths caused by CAD are sudden and unexpected. Many of these deaths happen to younger people in their 50s, 40s, or younger.

Defining Angina

When coronary artery disease progresses enough to significantly diminish the blood flow to heart tissue, it produces angina pectoris, which is commonly called angina. *Angina* typically is a discomfort felt in the chest, often beneath the breastbone (or sternum) or in nearby areas such as the neck, jaw, back, or arms.

- ✔ Individuals often describe the chest discomfort as a "squeezing sensation," "vicelike," "constricting," or " a heavy pressure on the chest." (In fact, the term *angina* comes from a Greek word that means "strangling" — a strangling pain.)

- ✔ Angina often is brought on by physical exertion or strong emotions and typically is relieved within several minutes by resting or using nitroglycerin.

- ✔ Some individuals may experience angina as a symptom different from chest discomfort or in addition to it. Shortness of breath, faintness, or fatigue may also be manifestations of angina, although if chest pain is absent, they may be called *anginal equivalents.*

- ✔ When chest pain occurs at rest, it usually is classified as *unstable angina.*

And just how do you pronounce the word? Some people say "an-*jī*-nuh" and others say "*an*-juh-nuh." Either is correct. Some cardiologists may be a little snobby about their preference (who, us?), but pay them no mind.

Understanding the causes of angina

You know how your muscles begin to scream when you run faster than your blood can carry adequate oxygen to them. The same thing may happen when the coronary arteries become so narrowed by atherosclerotic plaques that blood flow to the heart is inadequate to supply the heart muscle with the oxygen it needs. The temporary chest discomfort known as *angina* is your heart's way of getting your attention. It occurs when you ask your heart to work harder, and it therefore demands more blood — for instance, when you're walking briskly or running, climbing a hill or stairs, having sex, or doing housework or yardwork. Strong emotions such as fear or anger also can trigger an episode.

Considering angina's effect on the heart

Angina usually does not damage the heart. It is a temporary condition — the usual episode lasts only five to ten minutes. Chest discomfort makes you stop and rest, slowing the heart and lessening its demand for blood. Alternatively, most people with angina know to take a nitroglycerin tablet under the tongue when they have an angina attack. The nitroglycerin dilates the coronary arteries, enabling blood flow to the heart to increase.

Any discomfort that lasts longer that five to ten minutes or doesn't stop with rest may be a heart attack and needs to be treated as an emergency.

Diagnosing angina

An individual's own description of the discomfort he or she experiences provides the most important information leading to the diagnosis of angina. However, a number of tests also are used (see Chapter 11). Some of these tests can be conducted in your physician's office, but others require the resources of a hospital.

- ✔ **Electrocardiogram (ECG or EKG):** Tracings made by an ECG machine (to which a nurse hooks you up) during an episode of chest pain can show a number of characteristic changes that can help a physician make the diagnosis of angina.

- ✔ **Exercise tolerance testing (Exercise Stress Test):** The tracings of an ECG taken continuously as you exercise at increasing levels of exertion and as your heart rate increases can show changes that provide evidence of CAD and angina.

- ✔ **Nuclear stress testing:** This test may be required when the results of an individual's initial exercise tolerance test are equivocal (uncertain) or when the individual is not able to exercise. Special cameras take pictures of the heart when radioactive material (such as technetium, tetrofosmin, sestamibi, or thallium) is injected through a vein to assess the adequacy of blood flow. The stress portion of the test can be performed either with actual exercise or with a chemical stress agent (such as persantine or adenosine).

- ✔ **Stress echocardiogram:** An echocardiogram taken at rest and then during exercise or drug-simulated exercise can provide evidence of inadequate blood flow to the heart by showing images of the normal or abnormal motions of the heart muscle as it contracts.

- ✔ **High-speed CT scan:** High-speed computed tomography (CT) is an especially fast type of X-ray imaging that can provide a clear indication of the presence of calcium in the coronary arteries. The amount of calcification can help determine the presence and status of coronary artery disease.

✔ **Cardiac catheterization:** Cardiac catheterization, also called *cath* (slang) or *angiography,* often is used to make the final diagnosis of CAD when other tests have suggested that it is present. By taking actual pictures of the arteries when contrast material is injected into them, cardiac catheterization provides direct evidence whether narrowings are present and provides the physician with a road map that helps guide the patient and physician in determining the next steps in the treatment of CAD, whenever it is present.

Understanding two other types of angina

Although the most common form of angina results from the slow, progressive narrowing of the coronary arteries from coronary artery disease, two other rare forms of angina also may occur:

✔ **Variant angina,** or *Prinzmetal's angina,* which is named for Dr. Myron Prinzmetal, the cardiologist who first described this condition in 1959, occurs when the coronary arteries actually spasm, or contract suddenly. Although such episodes may occur in a normal coronary artery, spasm is most likely to occur where fatty plaque already is present. Treatment for this condition is similar to what is done for the more common form of angina, although a greater emphasis may be placed on medicines that decrease spasm (for example, calcium channel blockers, and nitrates — see "Treating unstable angina" later in the chapter).

✔ **Microvascular angina,** recently discovered, results from narrowing of tiny vessels in the heart while the major coronary arteries remain largely free of plaque. It is usually treated medically with common angina medications.

Distinguishing other causes of chest pain

All chest pain is not angina and does not involve the heart. Various conditions involving other structures in the chest can occasionally cause chest discomfort:

✔ Spasm of the esophagus

✔ Reflux of acid from the stomach

✔ Hiatal hernia

✔ Inflammation of the bones or cartilage of the chest wall or sternum

✔ Muscular pain from muscles of the chest wall, back, shoulders, or arms

In many of these instances, the characteristics of the pain distinguish it from angina. Pain typically is not coming from the heart if it

- ✔ Is extremely short in duration (lasting less than 10 seconds)
- ✔ Feels like it is on the surface of the chest wall rather than deep inside
- ✔ Is sharp, stabbing pain
- ✔ Is not associated with exertion

Treating angina

People who have angina typically can live comfortably for many years with this condition by finding out how to manage the symptoms and lower their risk factors for complications.

All patients with angina and underlying CAD need to be treated with risk-factor reduction and lifestyle modification to decrease the likelihood of complications from progressive narrowing of the coronary arteries. In addition, medications or surgery may be used as appropriate.

Risk factor reduction

Regardless of what other strategies your doctor employs, risk-factor reduction plays a critical role in managing the symptoms of angina and underlying CAD. As I discuss in Chapter 3, the critical factors include:

- ✔ Controlling high blood pressure
- ✔ Managing your cholesterol through improved nutrition and, in some instances, medications
- ✔ Managing your weight, if you're overweight
- ✔ Increasing the amount of physical activity in your life
- ✔ Quitting smoking, if you currently smoke

Controlling these risk factors is important for an overall heart-healthy lifestyle. I discuss risk factors fully in Parts IV and V of this book.

Lifestyle modifications

Developing angina can be a big blow emotionally. So big that patients often adopt an unrealistically gloomy perception of their prognosis. Actually, there's much you can do to adapt. Start with an open, frank discussion with your physician about how to use the following lifestyle modifications:

- Adjusting your approach to physical activity, leisure-time pursuits, vacation plans, eating habits, and other practices can help control and even reduce the symptoms of angina.

- Modifying strenuous activities that consistently and repeatedly produce angina can often be done by simple measures such as slowing your walking pace, strolling (not sprinting) to the car through the rain, vacuuming or raking more slowly, and so on.

- Avoiding strenuous activities that require heavy lifting, such as snow shoveling (unless you discuss it with your physician) is desirable.

- Adding slowly progressive exercise training, under your physician's supervision, can dramatically increase your ability to carry out enjoyable activities of daily living.

- Considering with your physician other interventions such as medication or surgery if your angina causes unacceptably severe modifications of your lifestyle can help. Quality of life is important!

Medical management

In conjunction with reducing risk factors and modifying certain activities, a variety of medicines can control the symptoms of angina. The medical management of angina is typically designed to diminish the demand for blood flow to the heart. The common medications include nitrates (particularly nitroglycerin), beta blockers, aspirin (particularly *enteric,* or coated, aspirin), and calcium antagonists.

Because all these medications also are used in the treatment of unstable angina, I discuss each class of medication in detail in the "Defining Unstable Angina" section.

Angioplasty and bypass surgery

Borrowing a concept from economics, the treatment of angina and unstable angina can be explained by the laws of supply and demand. Where medical management typically seeks to lower the heart's demand for blood flow, angioplasty and bypass surgery are designed to increase the supply of blood flow to the heart.

- In angioplasty, a balloon advanced by a catheter into the narrowed coronary artery is inflated to help open the artery. In many cases, a stent is also inserted to hold the artery open.

- In bypass surgery, a vein or artery from another part of the body is surgically grafted to a coronary artery to literally "bypass" a narrowing and restore blood flow.

For more information regarding these procedures, please see Chapter 16.

Knowing when chest pain is an emergency

People with coronary artery disease (CAD) and angina typically live with this problem for many years and discover how to manage it effectively with appropriate medicines and advice from their physicians. When angina pain changes in character, however, it can signal unstable angina or even heart attack. If you experience any of the following characteristics of chest discomfort, *you need to call 911 and be taken to a hospital immediately:*

✔ Pain or discomfort that is not relieved by three nitroglycerin tablets in succession, each taken five minutes apart

✔ Pain or discomfort that is worse than you have ever experienced before

✔ Pain or discomfort that is accompanied by fainting or lightheadedness, nausea, and/or cool clammy skin

✔ Pain or discomfort lasting longer than 20 minutes or that is very bad or worse than you have experienced before

If any of these symptoms occur, you need to call an ambulance and be taken immediately to a hospital. Under no circumstances should you drive yourself to the hospital (see Chapter 5).

Defining Unstable Angina

Although it typically results from underlying CAD and often is related to angina, unstable angina represents a significant turn for the worse. It usually is a medical emergency.

As the name suggests, *unstable angina* results when angina gets out of control. In unstable angina, the lack of blood flow and oxygen to the heart becomes acute and, therefore, very dangerous because the risk of complications such as heart attack is much greater.

Where stable angina has typical characteristics and predictable triggers, such as exertion or strong emotion, unstable angina is characterized by one or more of the following symptoms:

✔ Anginal discomfort at rest or when awakening from sleep

✔ A significant change in the pattern of the angina where it occurs with less exertion or is more severe than before

✔ A significant increase in the severity or frequency of angina

✔ New onset, or first experience, of anginal chest pain

If you experience any one of these characteristics, you must seek immediate medical attention.

Understanding the causes of unstable angina

The basic underlying CAD that causes angina also causes unstable angina. However, several additional elements also appear to contribute to turning angina into unstable angina:

✔ The plaque narrowing a coronary artery can crack open or rupture. When the body tries to heal the crack by forming a blood clot, this sudden narrowing can trigger a change from angina to unstable angina. When the clot blocks the artery entirely, a heart attack ensues. This process is depicted in Figure 4-2.

✔ In addition to the mechanical narrowing from the clot, substances released from the platelets may trigger the coronary artery to go into spasm, causing further narrowing and complications of the blockage that result in unstable angina.

Diagnosing unstable angina

If you have any of the symptoms described for unstable angina, you must be evaluated at the hospital.

If you've been diagnosed with CAD, use your previous experience as a guide in determining whether your symptoms suddenly have worsened. You need to call your physician whenever you experience any change in the circumstances related to your chest discomfort, the pattern of the chest discomfort, or the severity of the symptom.

Evaluating and responding to unstable angina in the emergency room

Because in its early manifestations unstable angina may be very difficult to distinguish from an acute heart attack, the procedures for evaluating both problems are similar in the emergency room. (See Chapter 5 on heart attacks.) It goes something like this:

✔ After you arrive at the hospital emergency room, physicians and nurses will evaluate you for signs of unstable angina.

✔ When a diagnosis of unstable angina seems probable, a number of medications may be administered to

• Prevent blood clots from forming in the coronary arteries.

• Increase the oxygen supply to your heart.

• Relieve pressure on the heart.

Communicating with physicians (and nurses) in the emergency room is of utmost importance so that you let them know whether your chest discomfort has been relieved.

✔ Your physician will take an electrocardiogram to help determine whether your heart is receiving adequate blood flow.

✔ Based on your past medical history, the nature of your chest discomfort, the electrocardiogram, and blood tests (in some instances), your emergency-room doctor will decide whether to keep you in the hospital. Even if your chest discomfort goes away, if your history strongly suggests unstable angina, admitting you to the hospital is imperative so that therapy is readily available and, in the event your chest discomfort recurs, medical staff can administer an electrocardiogram during an episode of chest discomfort to secure the diagnosis of unstable angina.

✔ If you're discharged home, your personal physician typically follows up in a day or two to evaluate you and perhaps order additional tests. *Note:* If you're discharged to home and your pain recurs, calling the ambulance and returning to the hospital is imperative. Don't be embarrassed or worried that you're being a bother — you're not.

Because angina of either variety can be difficult to diagnose in many instances, several visits with your physicians or the emergency room physicians may be required to be certain whether you have angina, and if so, whether it is stable or unstable.

Testing for unstable angina

In addition to the ECG, the tests that are helpful in both the diagnosis and the eventual treatment of unstable angina are the same as those discussed for angina: exercise tolerance test, stress echocardiogram, nuclear stress test, and cardiac catheterization (see the section "Diagnosing angina" earlier in this chapter).

Treating unstable angina

When tests reveal that you have narrowing of one, two, or three of the coronary arteries, your physician develops a plan for how best to treat your unstable angina. This plan may include the use of medicines, angioplasty (PCI), or coronary artery bypass surgery (CABG).

Medical therapy

A variety of medications that decrease the work of the heart or decrease the propensity of blood to clot at the sites of fatty plaques may be used to treat stable and unstable angina. The most common medications are

✔ **Nitrates:** Nitrates, particularly nitroglycerin, are valuable mainstays for treatment of angina and unstable angina. They relieve pressure on the heart and may also increase blood flow to the heart by causing the coronary arteries to dilate. Nitroglycerin often relieves discomfort quickly. Nitroglycerin/nitrates may come in the form of tablets or sprays that you put under the tongue, a pill that you take by mouth, a cream that you apply to your skin, or a patch that you wear on your skin. Some people may experience headache as a side effect.

✔ **Beta blockers:** These medications, another mainstay of treatment, decrease how hard the heart must work by lowering blood pressure and decreasing heart rate. In about 10 percent of individuals, side effects such as tiredness, dizziness, or depression can occur.

✔ **Calcium antagonists:** This class of medicines blocks calcium flow into the muscle cells of arteries and enables arteries to dilate. These medicines also are called *calcium channel blockers.* They typically are less effective than nitrates and beta blockers in angina treatment; however, calcium antagonists may be used in conjunction with them. Calcium antagonists are particularly useful when any significant degree of spasm of the coronary arteries is present.

✔ **Aspirin:** That's right, good old aspirin. Many people know that aspirin can relieve minor pain or fever, but they don't know that aspirin is important in treating angina and unstable angina because it helps prevent platelets from sticking to the walls of blood vessels and thereby contributing to any blood clot that may narrow or block off a coronary artery. Aspirin needs to be part of therapy for individuals with known or suspected CAD who haven't experienced any problems with bleeding. Research and experience show that using enteric, or coated, aspirin, which dissolves in the intestine, often helps lessen potential stomach irritation for individuals who are sensitive to aspirin.

✔ **Platelet receptor inhibitors:** This new category of drugs can enhance aspirin therapy by blocking the ability of platelets to stick to each other. These medicines, which typically are delivered intravenously in the hospital, may further help in the acute setting of unstable angina.

Angioplasty

An alternative to medical therapy that may be more appropriate to some patients with unstable angina is called *angioplasty, PTCA (percutaneous transluminal coronary angioplasty),* or *PCI (percutaneous coronary intervention).* This procedure uses the technique known as heart catheterization (see Chapter 16). In angioplasty, a catheter is inserted into an artery that is narrowed. Near the tip of this catheter is a small balloon that is inflated by a physician when the catheter reaches the blockage. When the balloon subsequently deflates, the blockage often is dilated enough for more blood to pass through, thus decreasing anginal discomfort. A stent (see Chapter 16) may also be inserted to keep the artery open.

Coronary artery bypass surgery

When the blockage of multiple coronary arteries is severe or the main branch of the left coronary artery is severely blocked, *coronary artery bypass surgery* (also called *coronary artery bypass grafting* or in medical slang, *CABG*) may be recommended as the most effective therapy. Surgery also is recommended when medical therapy and angioplasty don't control the symptoms of angina. During coronary artery bypass surgery, a piece of vein from the leg or an artery from the chest is grafted onto either side of a blocked coronary artery so that it bypasses the blockage (see also Chapter 16).

Fighting the good fight

Although coronary artery disease (CAD) and angina represent a significant health challenge to anyone diagnosed with them, there is no reason to surrender. A patient I'll call Mark sure didn't.

A driven, successful vice president of sales, Mark pushed himself hard — long days, snatched meals and snacks, lots of smokes, and no physical activity. At 48, he suffered a sudden heart attack. When he came to my office three weeks later, although he still was badly shaken, he also felt lucky to be alive. What could he do to turn his life around? Could he continue to prosper in his work without killing himself?

As we worked together on a plan for improving his health, he made a commitment to change. He quit smoking — a difficult task, but he did it. He cut excessive fat and calories out of his diet — at first because he had to, but then because he liked what he was eating and how he felt and looked. He started a walking program and worked up to jogging. He was such a changed man that a number of his salesmen began teasing him about his newfound commitment to health and fitness. One even called him a narcissist. "That made me mad," Mark said, "but then I thought, whoa. What's so bad about that? When I think about my life before, I remind myself of my dad — he dropped dead at 45 of a massive heart attack. So what's wrong with putting my health first? That way I'll be around to take care of my family, to excel in my work, and to enjoy my life!"

Working in an effective partnership with your physician, you too can combat, control, and tame this chronic condition.

Chapter 5

Understanding Heart Attacks

*T*he mere thought of a heart attack scares most people and with good reason: Nearly 1.5 million individuals suffer an acute heart attack every year in the United States alone. That's about one individual every 20 seconds. Worse yet, one-third of them die, and about one-half of these deaths occur within an hour of the event and usually are a result of cardiac rhythm problems associated with the heart attack.

Having a heart attack is all the more tragic because it often strikes individuals in their peak productive years. About 45 percent of heart attacks occur in individuals younger than age 65. Furthermore, of the Americans who die of coronary artery disease (CAD), the underlying condition that causes heart attacks, 29 percent of the women and 37 percent of the men are younger than 55.

Within this otherwise grim picture, however, is cause for some hope. The death rate from heart attacks decreased by about 25 percent during the last decade, and recent studies show that heart attacks are being diagnosed earlier and treated more effectively than ever before. And there's plenty of room for doctors to do even better.

In this chapter, I show you how to fight back against heart attacks, starting with educating yourself.

Defining a Heart Attack

A heart attack, known medically as a *myocardial infarction* (MI), occurs when one of the three coronary arteries that supply oxygen-rich blood to the heart muscle *(myocardium)* becomes severely or totally blocked, usually by a blood clot. When the heart muscle doesn't receive enough oxygenated blood, it begins to die. The severity of the heart attack depends on how much of the heart is injured or dies when it occurs.

When you think you're having a heart attack it's ever so critical to go immediately to a hospital where therapy can be initiated to save your heart muscle from dying. New clot-busting medicines, as well as procedures such as angioplasty, often can dissolve a clot that causes the heart attack, open the blood vessel, and save some or all of the heart muscle at risk. Although some of the heart muscle usually dies during a heart attack, the remaining heart muscle continues to function and often can compensate, to a very large degree, for the heart muscle that has died.

Understanding the causes of a heart attack

Heart attack almost always is caused when a blood clot forms at the site of an existing fatty plaque that has narrowed the coronary artery. Thus, individuals are at much higher risk for heart attack if they

✔ Have a history of CAD

✔ Have experienced previous bouts of angina

✔ Have suffered a previous heart attack

The blockage that triggers a heart attack usually is caused by an acute blood clot. Most *acute blood clots* occur when one of the plaques or fatty deposits on the artery walls cracks or ruptures (see Chapter 4). Other, much more rare causes of acute blockages in arteries supplying the heart include:

✔ Inflammation of the artery

✔ Spasm, or sudden contraction of one or more coronary arteries

✔ Certain blood-clotting abnormalities

✔ Severe spasm, acute blood clot, or other problem caused by cocaine use

Recognizing the symptoms of a heart attack

Different people experience the symptoms of a heart attack in different ways. However, typical symptoms include some or all of the following:

✔ A heavy chest pain or tightness, usually experienced in the front of the chest, beneath the sternum and often radiating to the left arm, left shoulder, or jaw

✔ Shortness of breath

✔ Nausea

✔ Sweating

✔ Clamminess, cool skin, pallor

✔ A feeling of general weakness or tiredness

In an individual who has angina, symptoms may be particularly difficult to differentiate from the chest discomfort of angina. (See Chapter 4.) However, when a heart attack is occurring, chest discomfort usually is more severe and may occur while the individual is at rest or less active than usual.

The signs of a heart attack often are subtle, particularly with individuals who have diabetes. Diabetics may not have the classic symptoms of chest, shoulder, or arm discomfort. Chest pain experienced by many women likewise may not present the classic symptoms.

 About two-thirds of the individuals who experience an acute heart attack also experience some warning symptoms in the weeks or days preceding the acute event. They often don't realize what the warning signs were until after the event — with keen hindsight. So work on your foresight. That way you'll know the warning signs of heart attack and take them seriously. (See the nearby sidebar "Experiencing heart attack warning signs? Call 911!")

Differentiating between heart attack and sudden cardiac arrest

 Although doctors often call sudden cardiac arrest "a massive heart attack," the two technically are not the same thing. A *massive heart attack* (myocardial infarction) results from a blockage of the coronary arteries. *Sudden cardiac arrest* is caused by ventricular fibrillation, an electrical malfunction in which the heart begins to quiver rapidly, instead of contracting and pumping blood regularly. Cardiac arrest strikes without warning. Because blood flow essentially stops, victims of cardiac arrest lose consciousness and die within minutes unless emergency help is available. (Chapter 6 discusses rhythm problems and cardiac arrest in detail.)

Many victims of sudden cardiac arrest have underlying CAD. Sudden cardiac arrest often (but not always) occurs in the setting of an acute heart attack. It can also occur from electrical malfunction when a heart attack is not involved.

Noting the complications associated with heart attacks

One of the key reasons for seeking medical therapy as early as possible for an acute heart attack is to enable the evaluations and therapies that will occur in the hospital (see the sections on emergency rooms and Coronary Care Units later in this chapter) to decrease possible complications such as the following:

✔ **Recurrent chest pain:** Recurrent or continued chest pain is one of the most dangerous aspects of an acute heart attack, because, as I note later in the section "Controlling cardiac pain," it indicates inadequate blood flow and often further damage to the heart. If your chest pain continues or recurs after you've been in the hospital, telling the health-care workers about it is important so they can take additional measures to alleviate chest pain and prevent further damage to the heart.

✔ **Arrhythmias:** An acute heart attack often damages the electrical system of the heart. That electrical system controls the heart's normal rhythm. Damaging it can result in rhythm problems, which also are called *arrhythmias* or *dysrhythmias.* When the electrical system goes entirely haywire, it may result in a very dangerous condition called *ventricular tachycardia,* which occurs when an abnormal electrical impulse causes the heart to beat so fast that it cannot pump out adequate blood. This condition can rapidly degenerate to *ventricular fibrillation,* which occurs when the heart simply quivers and produces no blood flow. Ventricular fibrillation must be immediately terminated by an electrical shock, or *defibrillation,* administered by a medical professional. (See Chapter 6 for more about rhythm disturbances.)

✔ **Heart failure:** When a heart attack severely damages the heart, either *acute* (sudden) *heart failure* or *chronic* (ongoing) *heart failure,* which is also called *congestive heart failure,* can ensue. A normal heart pumps out 75 percent to 80 percent of the blood in each chamber with each beat, but a heart damaged by a severe heart attack may pump only 15 percent to 20 percent, a condition that leads to heart failure. A number of medicines are available to treat acute and chronic heart failure. (Chapter 7 discusses the details of heart failure.)

✔ **Low blood pressure:** The reduced capacity of a heart damaged by an acute heart attack may result in low blood pressure, a condition called *hypotension.* When that happens blood pressure can get dangerously low, preventing adequate blood flow to coronary arteries and the rest of the body. Various medications and other interventions can be administered in the hospital to reverse the problem.

✔ **Disruption of a cardiac valve:** The four heart valves that control blood flow in, through, and out of the heart are operated by a series of muscles that can be damaged by an acute heart attack. When this happens, one or more valves may not be able to function normally. In this situation, torrential amounts of blood may flow back through the damaged valve, which in an otherwise undamaged condition would be closed. This condition, known as *valvular regurgitation,* can cause a serious problem during an acute heart attack. Medical and surgical options are available for treating this condition.

✔ **A rupture of the heart muscle:** When the part of the heart muscle that dies as a result of the heart attack is large or rendered very weak, this dead heart tissue can actually rupture or break open. This complication is catastrophic, because in many instances, the rupture is fatal. In other cases, a small hole in the heart can be repaired on an emergency basis by cardiac surgery.

✔ **Bleeding:** Although modern clot-busting medicines have revolutionized the treatment of heart attacks and saved many lives, they have one serious side effect: The same mechanism that enables them to dissolve clots in the coronary arteries can cause acute bleeding episodes elsewhere in the body. In the CCU, medical teams always are on the lookout for any evidence of bleeding, which can cause serious problems such as a stroke. Their goal is balancing the clot-busting benefits with prevention of excessive bleeding.

All these problems associated with heart attack can be diminished if the individual who's suffering the heart attack receives prompt medical therapy. I discuss these therapies in detail later in this chapter.

Taking Action — Immediately — for a Possible Heart Attack

Unfortunately, many people who are experiencing a heart attack either don't recognize symptoms or deny them. Don't let this scenario happen to you; it can be deadly. About half of all heart attack victims delay two hours or longer before deciding to get help. Doing so can be a serious or even fatal mistake, because delaying

✔ Significantly increases the risk of sudden death from heart rhythm problems in the early phases of a heart attack.

✔ Increases the likelihood that a significant amount of heart muscle will die, thus increasing the likelihood and extent of the heart attack, causing disability if the individual survives.

Timing is everything! If you or a loved one experiences any symptoms or warning signs of a heart attack, use the survival plan outlined in the next section and go immediately to a medical facility. Don't delay!

Experiencing heart attack warning signs? Call 911!

Coronary artery disease (CAD) is extremely common in men and women in the United States and particularly in individuals who are in their 40s and older. Even if you've never had a single sign of trouble, you need to call 911 and go straight to the hospital for prompt evaluation whenever you experience any of these warning signs (as described by the American Heart Association):

✔ Uncomfortable pressure, fullness, squeezing, or pain in the center of the chest lasting more than a few minutes

✔ Pain spreading to the shoulders, neck, or arms

✔ Chest discomfort with lightheadedness, fainting, sweating, nausea, or shortness of breath

Do not take a meeting. Do not put it off for an hour . . . *just call 911 and go!*

The following six-point survival plan, adapted from American Medical Association recommendations, can save your life. Take these steps if you or a loved one is experiencing the symptoms of a possible heart attack:

1. **Stop what you are doing, and sit or lie down.**

2. **If symptoms persist for more than two minutes, call your local emergency number or 911 and say that you may be having a heart attack.**

   Leave the phone off the hook so that medical personnel can locate your address in the event that you become unconscious.

3. **Take nitroglycerin, if possible.**

   If you have nitroglycerin tablets, take up to three pills under your tongue, one at a time, every five minutes, if your chest pain persists.

   If you don't have nitroglycerin, take two aspirin.

4. **Do not drive yourself (or a loved one) to the hospital if you think you are having a heart attack.**

   Ambulances have equipment and personnel who are trained to deal with individuals who are having a heart attack. Driving yourself or a loved one to the hospital is an invitation for a disaster.

5. **If the person's pulse or breathing stops, any individual trained in cardiopulmonary resuscitation (CPR) needs to immediately begin to administer it.**

If an automated external defibrillator (AED) is available, use it. Call 911 immediately, but do not delay instituting CPR or using an AED.

6. **When you arrive at the hospital emergency room, announce clearly that you (or your loved one) may be having a heart attack and that you must be seen immediately.**

    Don't be shy about it.

Diagnosing and Treating a Heart Attack in the Emergency Room

Modern emergency rooms have the medical teams and equipment needed to take immediate steps in determining whether you're having an acute heart attack and, if you are, to immediately start therapy that can reduce the severity of the heart attack and possibly even save your life.

When you arrive at the emergency room, teams of doctors and nurses take care of you immediately. They:

✔ Ask you questions about the nature of your symptoms while placing electrodes on your chest, arms, and legs so they can perform an electrocardiogram (ECG).

✔ Determine whether the ECG shows the characteristic patterns associated with acute heart attack, and if it does, they perform certain procedures immediately, such as administering clot-busting medicines to attempt to alleviate the blockage of the artery that is causing the heart attack. In many hospitals a patient experiencing a heart attack may be seen right away by a cardiologist and taken immediately to the cath lab for treatment.

✔ Find out (briefly) about your medical history to determine

   • The exact symptoms that you've either experienced or are currently experiencing

   • The duration of these symptoms

   • The severity of these symptoms

   • Your past medical history, and so on

✔ Quickly conduct a brief physical examination that focuses on the heart and lungs.

✔ Draw blood (simultaneously with the examination) to be sent to the laboratory to check for chemical markers that indicate damage to the heart.

The development of increasingly sensitive blood tests for such biomarkers as cardiac troponin and the MB fraction of creatine kinase (CK-MB) that occur in the presence of acute injury to heart muscle cells has enabled more precise treatment for individual patients. These tests can detect much smaller areas of injury than imaging techniques (see Chapter 11).

✔ Insert an intravenous line into a vein of the arm to enable prompt and efficient administration of medicines.

✔ Possibly make use of a defibrillator to administer electric current to restore (or shock) the heart back into a normal rhythm.

✔ Continually ask you about the level of chest discomfort you may be experiencing. Always answer as accurately as you can. (A heart attack is no time for silent bravery!)

✔ Administer medicines to diminish your discomfort and start treatment. These medicines include aspirin to decrease the clotting ability of platelets and beta blockers to slow the heart rate and lower your blood pressure. These medications have been proven to decrease complications of acute heart attack. Treatment with *thrombolytic therapy* (*thrombus* = clot, *lyse* = break up) also is started with intravenous clot-busting medicines.

All these procedures take place in rapid succession, with trained professionals calmly caring for you and reassuring you. Their goal is to create a calm atmosphere to diminish your anxiety.

Avoiding deadly excuses for delay

You've probably heard that getting treatment during the first "golden hour" after an accident gives trauma victims the best chance of survival and full recovery. The same is true of victims of biological accidents such as heart attacks. Using any of these common excuses for delay can be deadly:

✔ **How embarrassing if it's just heartburn.** And what if it isn't? Don't let a little embarrassment cost your life or your health.

✔ **I'm not sure whether my pain fits the warning signs.** The symptoms of heart attack vary from individual to individual and can be very vague. Let the physicians decide. It's their job, and they want to do it for you.

✔ **I'm too young to have a heart attack.** Heart attacks can and do happen at any age.

✔ **The pain's not that bad; I'll wait awhile and see whether it goes away.** Don't wait! Delaying significantly increases your risk of disabling damage and death.

✔ **Only men get heart attacks.** Whoa, ladies! Absolutely not! Women also suffer heart attacks, and their survival rate is not as good, in part, because they delay getting medical attention.

✔ **I'm as healthy as a horse — I can't be having a heart attack.** Denial never stopped a heart attack. For many victims, particularly younger people, heart attacks happen suddenly and without any noticeable warning signs.

Treating a Heart Attack in the Hospital Coronary Care Unit

If the initial evaluation in the emergency room either confirms the diagnosis of acute heart attack or raises a strong suspicion, you're admitted to the hospital or observed for 24 hours in the emergency department's *chest pain unit.* Your health-care team will provide much the same treatment measures in either setting.

If you're diagnosed with an acute heart attack, you're admitted to a specialized unit within the hospital called a *coronary care unit* (CCU). The CCU has specialized equipment and specially trained staff members who are able to continue your treatment and diagnose and quickly treat any complications that may occur from the acute heart attack. Your treatment typically contains a number of these elements:

- Continuing medical treatment to stabilize your condition, limit damage, and prevent complications.

- Continuous monitoring for potential complications such as heart rhythm problems, falling blood pressure, heart valve problems, continuing chest pain, or any other symptoms.

- Additional testing to confirm or rule out the diagnosis of acute heart attack and to determine the location and extent of the blockage. Testing also assesses the extent of injury to the heart muscle and the heart's ability to pump blood efficiently *(left ventricular function).*

Depending on the outcome of these procedures and tests, further procedures like angioplasty or coronary artery bypass surgery (see Chapter 16) may be performed to restore or maximize blood flow to the heart muscle and minimize the amount of muscle that is damaged or dies.

Considering typical medical treatments used in the CCU

Any or all of the treatment measures described in the sections that follow often are used to treat the early stages of a heart attack.

Preventing additional blood clots

Additional blood clots are a dangerous possibility for people who have just had a heart attack. The following medications help prevent more blood clots from occurring:

✓ **Aspirin,** as I mentioned in the section "Diagnosing and Treating a Heart Attack in the Emergency Room" earlier in this chapter, is used to decrease the "stickiness" of platelets and thus lessen their ability to continue to form blood clots within the coronary arteries.

✓ **Anticoagulants,** or blood thinners, also protect against the tendency of additional blood clots forming either in the coronary arteries or within one of the heart's chambers near the damaged area of muscle.

✓ **Platelet receptor inhibitors** are new medicines that act in conjunction with aspirin to further keep platelets from sticking together.

✓ **Statins,** which help reduce cholesterol, may also be administered (see Chapter 14 for more about cholesterol).

Controlling cardiac pain

Pain management is important in treating an acute heart attack, because cardiac pain is a marker for continued damage to the fragile cells of the heart muscle. Controlling pain indicates decreasing damage, because pain is a marker of continuing damage. Pain management typically is accomplished with a combination of medicines such as pain relievers, nitrates, and beta blockers.

✓ **Pain relievers,** also called *analgesics,* can be used during the acute phase of a heart attack. Morphine is probably the most commonly used.

✓ **Nitrates,** such as nitroglycerin, increase blood flow through coronary arteries and decrease the work of the heart.

✓ **Beta blockers** decrease pressure on the heart and slow the heart rate, both of which decrease the demand from the heart muscle for oxygen.

✓ **Oxygen** improves the supply of oxygenated blood to the heart muscle. This is typically delivered through an oxygen mask or an oxygen tube that's placed in the nose.

Looking at typical tests given in the CCU

In the CCU, monitoring is continuous and medications are given to decrease pain and limit the size of the heart attack. The additional tests in the list that follows likewise may be conducted in the CCU.

✓ **Electrocardiograms (ECG)** are typically taken at least every eight hours to check for evidence of the extent of the heart attack and provide an early warning for some of the potential complications of a heart attack. You also undergo continuous ECG monitoring to assess the electrical activity of the heart.

✔ **Physical examinations** are usually performed at least every six hours to check for complications of the heart attack and assess your lungs to find out whether any fluid buildup has occurred, which decreases the oxygen supply to the heart and further complicates the heart attack.

✔ **Echocardiograms** are ultrasound tests that are performed on some patients to assess how well their hearts are working and look for any complications of a heart attack that may have occurred. This test may also help determine whether chest pain is being caused by something other than a lack of blood flow to the heart *(ischemia)*.

✔ **Coronary angiography, or heart catheterization,** often is conducted within the first two or three days following an acute heart attack or unstable angina to help doctors assess the degree of narrowing in the coronary arteries and the effectiveness of any clot-busting medicine that was administered.

Noting other procedures that may be needed

Doctors check the severity of the narrowing of the coronary arteries not only in the area affected by the heart attack but also throughout the coronary arterial system. Your physicians may recommend angioplasty or bypass surgery to help maintain or restore adequate blood flow to the heart for the longer term.

Recuperating from a Heart Attack

A typical stay in a CCU usually lasts two to three days for an uncomplicated heart attack. If heart attack has been ruled out, a stay in the chest pain unit or CCU may be for only 24 hours. But if complications occur, the stay in the CCU can be extended to four or five days or even longer.

After you've been stabilized and the acute events surrounding your heart attack have been treated, you enter what most large hospitals call a step-down unit. Your stay in the step-down unit will be for the next four to six days, or until you complete your recovery and begin rehabilitation from the heart attack.

The rehabilitation process starts in the hospital and takes place during the next few months after you're discharged from the hospital. The rehabilitative steps that you take in the hospital include

✔ Changing over to medications that can be taken orally.

✔ Working with your physician and trained cardiac rehabilitation special-ists to assess your condition and start treatment of risk factors for heart disease that may be present. (Yes, it's back to school for you.)

✔ Beginning a progressive increase in physical activity, starting with slow walking initially in your room, followed by walking in the hospital hallway.

Prior to discharge from the hospital, many individuals also may undergo a low-level exercise tolerance test on a treadmill to determine the degree of their functional recovery and to guide the physicians in prescribing addi-tional, necessary procedures. Others instead may take a symptom-limited exercise tolerance test a few weeks later.

In addition to the physical and medical issues, almost every patient undergoes a spectrum of emotional responses to acute heart attack. These responses vary from extreme anxiety during the actual event to depression and remorse after-ward. The good news: The vast majority of individuals who survive a heart attack go on to lead long and productive lives. In fact, 88 percent of heart attack survivors younger than 65 can return to work within three months. The process of cardiac rehabilitation is so important that I devote all of Chapter 18 to it.

Chapter 6

Beating Out of Sync: Arrhythmias

• •

In This Chapter

▶ Defining rhythm problems in the heart's electrical system

▶ Understanding specific rhythm problems

▶ Diagnosing cardiac rhythm problems

▶ Treating rhythm problems

• •

Day in and day out, the beat goes on — the heartbeat, that is — and all that beating depends on the heart's electrical system. Infinitely subtle and wonderfully specialized, the heart's electrical system enables the heart to accelerate smoothly from 40 to 50 beats up to 200 beats per minute and then decelerate back with nary a hitch. But when this electrical system suffers from some insult, such as lack of blood flow to the heart, it can start causing problems.

In this chapter, I sort through the seemingly bewildering causes and conditions that can result in cardiac rhythm problems, called *arrhythmias*. I also tell you when to worry and when not to.

Defining Arrhythmias

Cardiac *arrhythmias,* also called cardiac *dysrhythmias,* are irregularities or abnormalities in the beating of the heart. Arrhythmias are surprisingly common. They can arise in a wide variety of settings and can range from totally insignificant to life-threatening. In fact, if everyone were hooked up to a 24-hour, continuous electrocardiogram (such as the Holter monitor that I discuss in Chapter 11), you'd find that everyone experiences a few extra heartbeats and a few skipped heartbeats. Technically, all these extra and skipped heartbeats are cardiac arrhythmias. Yet, for the vast majority, these minor irregularities carry absolutely no health consequences.

More severe cardiac arrhythmias, however, can be deadly. Consider that

▶ More than 40,000 individuals in the United States die each year from a primary rhythm problem.

✔ Rhythm problems are a contributing cause of death in about 25 percent of all deaths each year in the United States.

✔ More than 4 million people are admitted to hospitals every year with a rhythm problem as at least part of their initial symptoms.

Understanding your heart's electric company

What does electricity have to do with the causes of arrhythmia? Everything. In the final analysis, all cardiac rhythm problems relate to the underlying electrical activity that drives the heart and tells it when to beat and to the interaction between this electrical activity and the heart's anatomy. But before getting into what causes these electrical problems, reviewing and expanding your understanding of the heart's electric company is necessary.

As I discuss in Chapter 2, the cardiac electrical system is an exquisite grouping of cells and fibers that uses electrical impulses to tell the heart when to contract. You can follow the route of these electrical impulses, using the schematic drawing of this system in Figure 6-1. (Don't worry, it's much easier to follow than the wiring schematic in your car manual.)

A small group of cells high up in the right atrium controls the rhythm of the heart. This group of cells is called the *sinus node,* or *sinoatrial node.* Acting as the heart's pacemaker, these cells spontaneously discharge an electrical impulse that is carried through the atrium and down to another node located at the intersection of the atria and the ventricles. Not surprisingly, this second node is called the *atrioventricular node,* or *AV node.*

Behaving like a traffic cop, the AV node receives electrical signals from the sinus node, slows them down, and makes sure that the proper number of signals alerts the ventricles to contract.

Below the AV node are two more specialized bundles of muscle fibers located in the *septum,* the muscular wall that separates the two ventricles. These specialized bundles function as pathways carrying electrical signals to contract to all of the cells in both ventricles. (If you've just got to know, these pathways are called the *His-Purkinje system.*)

Whenever this primary electrical system has problems, the heart actually has an emergency backup system. If the sinus node doesn't fire, other cells in the electrical system, such as the AV node or the His-Purkinje system can send a spontaneous signal to the heart muscle cells to contract. But there's a catch. At each lower level of command, the rate of the electrical impulse slows, so the heart beats or contracts more and more slowly.

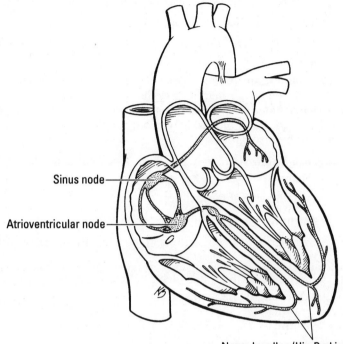

Sinus node

Atrioventricular node

Figure 6-1:
The heart's
electrical
system.

Nerve bundles (His-Purkinje system)

In addition to its own internal electrical system, the heart also is influenced by the body's ultimate electrical system — the brain and central nervous system. You might say that the cardiac electrical system is *networked,* to use a modern concept. Working at its best, this network creates the ultimate flexibility for changes in cardiac rhythm that respond to the heart's particular needs. The central nervous system, for example, orders the heart to speed up when you start to run and to slow down when you rest or sleep.

Looking at what happens when the heart's electric company goes haywire

When anything disturbs or interrupts the normal functioning of the heart's electrical system, problems with cardiac rhythm result. A variety of underlying conditions, which often are interrelated, can cause cardiac rhythm problems. These include

✔ **Problems related to the electrical system itself,** including:

• The sinus node losing its ability to trigger the electrical impulses or triggering them erratically.

- Cells that normally fire by themselves losing their ability to do so.

- The AV node losing its ability to direct the signal.

- The signal to beat originating someplace other than the sinus node.

✔ **Lack of blood flow to living tissues of the electrical system,** such as that produced by coronary artery disease (CAD) including heart attack. The lack of blood flow can cause abnormal rhythm patterns or conduction blocks or heart blocks, in which the signal encounters difficulty even getting through.

✔ *Congenital abnormalities,* **problems that people are born with,** such as:

- Certain valve abnormalities

- Abnormal heart chambers

- Extra electrical connections in the heart that produce *SVTs,* fast heart rhythms

- Calcium growth around electrical system cells

✔ **The effect of underlying disease states or conditions,** such as:

- CAD

- Coronary valve disease or heart failure

- Stress

- Flu — ever wonder why your heart beats fast when you have a fever?

✔ **The results of things you do to yourself,** such as using

- Caffeine (Has an extra cup of coffee ever caused your heart to race?)

- Tobacco

- Alcohol

- Diet pills

- Cough and cold medicines

- Illegal drugs such as cocaine and amphetamines

Recognizing the symptoms of cardiac arrhythmias

The symptoms of cardiac rhythm problems are as diverse as the problems themselves. They also range from inconsequential to life-threatening.

✔ **Palpitations:** Probably the least worrisome of symptoms, *palpitations* describe a variety of uncomfortable sensations of your heartbeat, such as the sensation that your heart is missing or skipping a beat. To some people, palpitations may feel like a fluttering in the chest. In and of themselves, these skipped or missed beats aren't terribly worrisome. However, when multiple skipped beats occur in succession, they can lead to serious problems.

✔ **A racing or pounding heart:** Although these symptoms can arise from strong emotion or exercise, if they occur while you're at rest, they may indicate a significant rhythm problem.

✔ **Lightheadedness or dizziness:** Everybody becomes lightheaded or dizzy every now and then, but if these symptoms are not one-time passing events, you need to have your doctor check out possible causes, which include heart rhythm problems

✔ **Passing out:** Unlike fainting spells in which faintness may come on a bit gradually — with the world graying out and with your body going sweaty or clammy — fainting spells caused by rhythm problems tend to be sudden. Anyone who experiences a sudden fainting spell, or more than one episode of what seems to be an ordinary fainting spell, needs to seek medical attention to determine the underlying problem.

✔ **Cardiac collapse:** This most severe rhythm problem in some instances can be treated effectively with cardiopulmonary resuscitation (CPR) or automated external defibrillation (AED). Cardiac collapse (also called cardiac arrest) is without a doubt a life-threatening emergency: Approximately 95 percent of the people who suffer sudden cardiac arrest die before they reach the hospital. Quick use of CPR and AED can double their chances of survival. Anyone who survives such an episode requires advanced electrical diagnostic techniques in the hands of a skilled cardiologist trained in the subspeciality of electrophysiology.

Taking a Look at Specific Rhythm Problems

Just like people, rhythm problems come in different shapes and sizes. In an attempt to lend some order to this complex field, cardiologists typically classify rhythms according to their anatomic point of origin. Very broadly, rhythm problems can be characterized as arising from structures in the atria, including the sinus node and the AV node, located between the right atrium and ventricle, and from structures in the ventricles.

Rhythm problems that arise in the atria usually are less dangerous than the ones that arise in the ventricles, because the atria act as booster pumps, compared to the ventricles, which are the main power source for circulating blood throughout the body. As a consequence, any rhythm problems that impede the ventricles' ability to do their work can lead to serious trouble.

Considering rhythm problems arising in the atria

These rhythm problems typically are a result of the electrical system causing the heart to beat too fast, a symptom known as *tachycardia;* too slow, *bradycardia;* or chaotically, *fibrillation.*

Sinus tachycardia

Although the heart must be able to beat fast when you exercise or exert yourself, a fast heartbeat when you're at rest can cause problems, particularly if you have any narrowing of your coronary arteries. Among the variety of situations that can lead to *sinus tachycardia* are fever, certain endocrine abnormalities (such as an elevated thyroid level), anxiety, and pain.

Bradycardia

To some degree, a slow heartbeat may actually be desirable. For example, a trained athlete often has a heart rate in the high 40s or low 50s when at rest. However, in cardiology, any resting heart rate of less than 60 is called *bradycardia.* Bradycardia becomes dangerous when the electrical signal generated by the sinus node is so slow that the heart doesn't beat often enough to pump adequate blood. When that happens, treating the slow heart rate either with medication or in some instances with a pacemaker may be necessary.

Atrial flutter

When lovers say that their hearts are fluttering, they're describing a pleasing sensation. However, the sensation isn't so great when an atrium starts to flutter. In an *atrial flutter,* a very rapid, regular electrical signal (which is not effectively transmitted to the ventricles) causes a very rapid heartbeat. Correcting this condition requires either medication or *cardioversion,* a therapy that uses a carefully controlled electrical current to shock the atrium back into better behavior. (For more details about cardioversion, see Chapter 11.)

Atrial fibrillation

Atrial fibrillation occurs when electrical signals are chaotic and muscles of the atria quiver rather than contract. The electrical impulses also reach the ventricles very erratically, thus producing an erratic heartbeat. This condition is common in individuals who have heart disease and can be caused by a variety of conditions including CAD artery disease, hypertension, and an elevated thyroid level.

Atrial fibrillation, by itself, is not immediately life-threatening. But because the atria are not contracting effectively, they can gather clots that can pass through the heart and into either the brain or the lungs. If a clot travels to the brain, it typically results in a stroke. A clot in the lungs can cause a very serious condition called *pulmonary embolism*. (For more information about these conditions, see Chapter 9.)

Because of the possible outcomes, treating atrial fibrillation aggressively is important. Treatment may include medications and/or cardioversion. In addition to medicines to control the heart rate, all patients who have atrial fibrillation must take blood-thinning medicines (anticoagulants) to lower the risk of blood clots generated in the atria being thrown to the brain or lungs.

Other atrial arrhythmias

Several other rhythm irregularities or problems arise in the atria.

- ✔ *Sinus arrhythmia* refers to cyclical changes in heart rate during breathing. Although more common in children, it also occurs in adults. This irregular rhythm pattern, however, is not considered a problem and requires no treatment.

- ✔ *Premature atrial contractions* (PAC), an early beat in the atria, cause the heart to beat before the regular beat.

- ✔ Two conditions involving a series of early atrial beats, called *supraventricular tachycardia* (SVT) and *paroxysmal atrial tachycardia* (PAT) speed up the heart rate. In PAT, the fast heart rate begins and ends suddenly.

- ✔ In a condition called Wolff-Parkinson-White Syndrome, abnormal electrical pathways between the atria and ventricles enable the electrical signal to bounce back and forth between the atria and ventricles creating a very rapid heart beat.

Considering rhythm disturbances arising in the ventricles

Rhythm disturbances similar to those in the atria originate in the ventricles. However, as I already indicated in "Taking a Look at Specific Rhythm Problems," because these rhythm problems affect the main pumping chambers of the heart, they usually are more significant or dangerous than those affecting the atria. The sections that follow detail some of the common rhythm problems that can arise in the ventricles.

Ventricular premature contractions

Ventricular premature contractions (also called VPCs or PVCs) can occur when a small grouping of cells in the ventricle generates an abnormal electrical signal. This extraneous signal causes the heart to beat prematurely and takes one or more beats out of the normal sequence. Individuals often do not even recognize these premature beats, but if they do, they usually experience the sensation of skipping a beat or having an extra one.

VPCs can occur in anyone but are more common in individuals who have underlying CAD. Occasional VPCs typically are not worrisome. But VPCs pose a danger when they start grouping together or occurring more frequently, because they may stimulate or trigger much more serious cardiac problems, such as ventricular tachycardia or ventricular fibrillation.

Ventricular tachycardia

Ventricular tachycardia occurs when continuous extra heartbeats originate from an abnormal group of cells in the ventricle. If sustained for any length of time, this condition is very dangerous, because when the ventricles are in this racing rhythm, your heart cannot pump adequate amounts of blood. When its onset is sudden or acute, ventricular tachycardia requires an electrical shock to the heart using a defibrillator to convert it back into a normal rhythm. To prevent further episodes of this dangerous rhythm, you either start taking anti-arrhythmic medicines or have a permanent defibrillator implanted in the chest to deliver a small electric shock directly to your heart whenever ventricular tachycardia occurs.

Ventricular fibrillation

Ventricular fibrillation is the most dangerous cardiac arrhythmia. Ventricular fibrillation occurs following an episode of ventricular tachycardia. It, in fact, usually is triggered by ventricular tachycardia. In ventricular fibrillation, the ventricle *fibrillates,* or quivers, and does not adequately contract to generate oxygenated blood flow to the working heart or other organs. This form of arrhythmia is a medical emergency that requires immediate electrical shock to try to jolt the heart back into a normal rhythm. Failure to stop ventricular fibrillation typically results in death.

Passing the beat on poorly: Conduction problems

In addition to rhythm problems, abnormalities can occur in the actual conduction of electrical impulses throughout the heart. These conduction problems can affect not only various components of the heart's specialized electrical system but also individual cardiac cells.

The most severe of these conditions are known as *heart blocks,* or *conduction blocks.* Heart blocks describe the inability of electrical impulses from the AV node to reach the ventricles in a timely fashion, and they result in inadequate blood flow. Heart blocks may be caused by heart disease, certain drug toxicities, electrolyte problems, or trauma, but they do not describe blocked flow of blood to the heart. Think of a heart block as the AV node not functioning properly. Heart blocks can delay each signal, block parts of the signals, or block all signals from reaching the ventricles. When a complete heart block occurs, the ventricles' backup system initiates the heartbeat, but the rate is slow and insufficient. The most effective treatment for a severe heart block condition is a temporary or permanent cardiac pacemaker.

Diagnosing Cardiac Rhythm Problems

Cardiologists rely on a wide variety of techniques, ranging from very simple to extremely complex, to help diagnose underlying rhythm disturbances. I describe these techniques more fully in Chapters 10 and 11, but here are some of the ways they are used to diagnose rhythm problems.

✔ **History:** A detailed history of exactly what symptoms you experience and under what circumstances they occur is extremely valuable in diagnosing an underlying cardiac rhythm problem. As I indicate in the previous section, symptoms may range from palpitations to fainting or cardiac collapse.

When you're experiencing minor rhythm problems, such as palpitations, taking your own pulse during an episode, thus trying to further characterize what is happening to your heart rate, is a good idea. Your physician may ask you to tap out the rhythm during an office visit.

✔ **Physical examination:** Your physician conducts a complete physical examination with an emphasis on the cardiovascular system. In addition to listening to your heart, your physician may perform other procedures, such as pressing on one of the arteries in your neck, a technique that often slows down the heart and may provoke a rhythm problem that may cause you to faint. Your physician may also ask you to perform a little mild exercise during an exam.

✔ **Electrocardiogram (ECG):** The next step after the history and physical examination is an electrocardiogram. Because the ECG traces electrical impulses of the heart, it provides an excellent indication of many of the underlying problems that can result in rhythm disturbances. An ECG also can pick up abnormalities in the conduction of electrical impulses that have not caused any symptoms. These abnormalities, which usually require no treatment, may be insignificant or they may be subtle indicators of potential future problems that your physician may want to keep an eye on.

✔ **Exercise tolerance testing:** Sometimes arrhythmias that are provoked when the heart is going faster can be determined by performing exercise tolerance testing. In this situation, your physician looks either for rhythm problems that are stimulated by the heart going faster or for inadequate blood flow to the heart when exercise makes your heart work harder at faster speeds.

✔ **Long-term electrocardiographic monitoring:** Doctors often ask their patients to wear an electrocardiographic monitoring system to detect and record underlying heart rhythm problems. You may even be asked to wear an event monitor that is activated (either by you or automatically) when a rhythm disturbance occurs or a 24-hour Holter monitor, which I describe in Chapter 11. Both enable you to function normally during monitoring.

✔ **Electrophysiological studies:** Electrophysiological studies, also called EPS, have grown in sophistication and diagnostic use during the last 25 years. This procedure is similar to a cardiac catheterization. However, in this case, catheters with electrical monitoring sensors are passed into various chambers of the heart in an attempt either to monitor a rhythm problem or to stimulate one so that a precise treatment can be determined. Electrophysiological studies are absolutely necessary whenever you've been resuscitated from a cardiac collapse. EP studies may also be highly relevant when you've fainted and the underlying cause may be cardiac in nature. In addition, EP studies may be useful if you're having persistent and dangerous rhythm problems that cannot be managed with medications.

Treating Rhythm Problems

As I've hinted in the discussions of types of rhythm problems, a wide variety of treatments are available. As you look over the following sections, which describe those treatments, remember that in all therapies your active participation and commitment are critical to success.

Using lifestyle measures

As I note earlier in the section "Recognizing the Symptoms of Cardiac Arrhythmias," palpitations are the most common symptom of arrhythmia and may be caused by or made worse by practices such as drinking too many caffeinated beverages (coffee, tea, and many soft drinks), consuming too much alcohol, not effectively treating stress, or not obtaining adequate rest. Changing any or all of these lifestyle measures often can make palpitations disappear.

Treating underlying illnesses

If an underlying illness, such as a fever, pain, anxiety, or endocrine problem, causes a rhythm problem, treating the underlying condition is essential to treating the rhythm problem. Thus, it is important for your physician to explore and treat any underlying conditions as part of the therapy for your cardiac rhythm problems.

Prescribing medications

A bewildering variety of medications are available to treat cardiac arrhythmias. Likewise, the manner by which these medications are administered can be very complex. So if you have a serious rhythm problem, your personal physician probably will consult with a cardiologist who is skilled in the use of these medications.

Depending on its mechanism of action and exactly how it works within the cardiac electrical system, each medication falls into one of four major classifications. Not surprisingly, a numbering system denotes these four classes. If you are taking an anti-arrhythmic drug, you're taking a Class 1, Class 2, Class 3, or Class 4 medication. Your physician isn't likely to specify which particular classification your medication fits within. However, your doctor is guided by this broad scheme when selecting the proper medication for your specific cardiac rhythm problem from among 30 to 40 anti-arrhythmic drugs that are available.

Employing electrical therapy

In the same way that cardiologists who specialize in heart catheterization are known as *plumbers,* cardiologists who specialize in treating cardiac rhythm problems with electrical therapy are known as *electricians.* Electrician is a term of endearment for these men and women, who possess a highly specialized knowledge that can prove lifesaving for many cardiac patients. Four different kinds of electrical therapy are outlined in the sections that follow.

Cardioversion

You can describe this form of treatment by saying it takes one to fix one. Because the heart is an electrical system, the skilled application of an external source of electricity can jolt the heart back into its normal rhythm. This process is called *cardioversion.*

During cardioversion therapy, the patient usually is mildly sedated (of course, in an emergency, time is not taken for sedation). Two electrical paddles are applied to the chest wall at the level of the heart and an electrical current is passed through the heart. This shock causes the electrical system to reboot itself and often pop back into the normal sinus rhythm that is desirable.

Cardioversion can effectively treat various cardiac arrhythmias, including atrial fibrillation, atrial flutter, ventricular tachycardia, and ventricular fibrillation. Cardioversion, also called *defibrillation,* is literally a lifesaver in emergencies when acute ventricular tachycardia and ventricular fibrillation threaten immediate death because the heart is not putting out any oxygenated blood. Modern cardioversion or defibrillation equipment is capable of sensing underlying cardiac rhythm and applying exactly the right amount of shock at exactly the right time to maximize the likelihood of converting the heart back into its normal rhythm.

Automatic implantable defibrillators

Automatic implantable defibrillators, also known as implantable cardioverter-defibrillators (ICDs), perform a particularly effective type of cardioversion, and their development has provided new leases on life to patients with serious ventricular rhythm problems. When implanted inside the chest, the device monitors the heart's rhythm and quickly administers an electrical shock as needed to correct any serious arrhythmias. Although when the defibrillator goes off, or fires, patients feel a sensation as if they've been bopped in the chest, they typically don't mind receiving that kind of wakeup call. They say it's certainly preferable to the alternative.

Pacemaker therapy

Pacemakers typically are used when the heart has very slow rhythm, particularly as a result of conduction blocks. Modern cardiac pacemakers can sequentially pace both the atria and the ventricles to generate an effective cardiac output. These pacemakers are able to sense the heart's own rhythm and kick into action only when that rhythm slows to a certain point. Advances in electronic design and battery power also have enabled pacemakers to be made smaller and last for ten or more years between battery changes. And, to the delight of those who rely on them, modern pacemakers are not sensitive to microwave ovens and the like.

Surgical therapy

Surgical procedures that treat cardiac arrhythmias vary from techniques aimed at destroying abnormal electrical cells to prevent them from making the heart beat too fast to implanting defibrillators and pacemakers.

Most advanced surgical procedures require an operating room and surgeons skilled in cardiac rhythm problems, a specialized catheterization laboratory devoted to electrical abnormalities and correcting them, or both. This laboratory is called an *electrophysiology* laboratory, and the cardiologists who specialize in this area are called *electrophysiologists.*

Electrophysiological techniques can be used to evaluate and diagnose a wide variety of rhythm problems and to administer catheter ablation to cauterize the areas of muscle responsible for abnormal electrical activity and restore normal electrical activity.

Chapter 7

When the Pump Falters: Heart Failure

For many folks, *heart failure* conjures up an image of a heart that suddenly stops or a heart that's totally ruined. Relax. Neither image is accurate. Heart failure, which often is called *congestive heart failure* (CHF), is the term cardiologists use to describe the condition of a heart that is no longer able to adequately pump blood to meet the body's needs. You can experience varying degrees of heart failure, and many factors contribute to this condition. Heart failure always is serious but not instantly fatal. You can do many things to maximize the quality and length of life if you or a loved one is diagnosed with heart failure. Moreover, I describe plenty of things in this chapter that you can do to prevent heart failure from developing in the first place.

Defining Heart Failure

Heart failure occurs when the heart no longer adequately pumps blood to the lungs and throughout the body. It usually is a slow process that takes place during a period of years. Underlying conditions, such as coronary artery disease (CAD), leakage from one of the heart valves, or various diseases of the heart muscle itself usually cause heart failure. The heart initially compensates for small decreases in its ability to pump by doing the following:

✔ Enlarging (*dilatation*) to enable more blood into its pumping chambers

✔ Thickening the muscle walls (*hypertrophy*) to strengthen the pump and enable it to exert more force during its contraction to move more blood

> ✔ Beating faster to make up for decreased volume or power (like trying to pitch more, but smaller, pails of water on a fire)

The heart may try to compensate in these ways for years before you notice any symptoms. But when these mechanisms ultimately fail, significant heart failure occurs. By then, compensatory mechanisms often have become part of the problem.

How serious heart failure is depends on how much pumping capacity the heart has lost. A normal heart discharges about 75 percent of the blood in the main pumping chambers with each contraction, or beat. Heart failure often occurs when the amount of blood ejected per beat, called the *ejection fraction*, drops below 50 percent, and when the ejection fraction falls below 40 percent heart failure ensues. Even so, many people can survive for many years with ejection fractions of only 20 percent to 30 percent, or sometimes even 15 percent.

However, the greater the loss of pumping capacity, the more likely you are to suffer a number of complications. All forms of heart failure are serious health problems that require medical treatment. Taking care of yourself, seeing your physician regularly, and paying scrupulous attention to recommended treatments are important steps you can take to improve your chances of living longer. Fortunately, significant advances have occurred during the last five years in the medical profession's knowledge of heart failure and in the treatments that are available.

Looking at different types of heart failure

Heart failure is not just one disease; it's actually a way of describing a group of conditions and symptoms that occur when any of a number of problems prevents the heart from pumping enough blood. Therefore, you can look at heart failure in several ways. The most common (described in the following list) are which side of the heart is most affected and which part of the cardiac cycle is most affected.

> ✔ **Left heart failure:** When the left ventricle of the heart cannot adequately pump blood out to the body, the blood begins to back up into the lungs. In this form of heart failure, which usually is called *congestive heart failure,* fluid seeps out of the backed-up blood vessels and into the small airways of the lungs, making them congested (hence the name). Shortness of breath is the most pronounced symptom of this condition. Several underlying conditions, which I discuss in the sections that follow, can contribute to left heart failure.

> ✔ **Right heart failure:** In right heart failure, the right ventricle isn't pumping adequately. The most obvious symptom is a buildup of fluid in the legs and ankles, a condition of swelling called *edema.* Right heart failure usually occurs as an ultimate result of left heart failure. However, people

with severe lung disease can also experience right heart failure, because the right heart isn't able to generate enough pressure to pump blood through a diseased pair of lungs. This last condition is called *cor pulmonale* (see Chapter 9).

✔ **Systolic heart failure:** In this condition, the heart doesn't eject enough blood during its contraction, or its *systole*. Symptoms of systolic heart failure typically include lung congestion and swelling (or edema) in the legs.

✔ **Diastolic heart failure:** In this condition, the heart doesn't relax between contractions, or its *diastole*. As a result, not enough blood can enter the pumping chamber, which in turn causes fluid to gather (edema) in the abdomen and legs, a symptom that's typical of diastolic heart failure.

Identifying the groups that heart failure affects most

Although heart failure is a very serious medical condition for anyone, some people tend to suffer more complications from heart failure than others, including:

✔ **The aged:** The prevalence of heart failure most commonly increases with age. Men and women older than age 70 who have heart failure are significantly more likely to die from it than younger individuals.

✔ **Men:** Although men and women tend to get heart failure in comparable numbers, men tend to suffer more problems and don't survive as long after diagnosis as women. Researchers don't totally understand the reasons for the discrepancy.

✔ **African Americans:** Heart failure occurs more often (by about 25 percent) and is more often fatal in men and women who are African American than in White Americans. Although the reasons why heart failure is more prevalent and deadly among African Americans are unclear, at least two factors that undoubtedly contribute are the greater incidence among African Americans of hypertension and diabetes, which often underlie heart failure, and a pattern of less timely access to health care.

Understanding the Causes of Heart Failure

Anatomy is destiny, I often say. Anatomically, the heart is a pump. Any condition that significantly compromises the heart's ability to function as a pump, overloads the pump, or restricts it ability to fill up leads to heart failure.

Directly damaging the heart muscle

By far, the most common causes of heart failure are events or conditions that damage the muscle of the heart itself, the *myocardium*. And what cardiac culprits most frequently damage the heart muscle?

- ✔ **Heart attack:** The muscle damage and scarring caused by a heart attack can weaken the heart's pumping strength. (See Chapter 5 for details about heart attack.)

- ✔ **Myocarditis:** This uncommon condition is an acute inflammation of the heart muscle (*myo* = heart, *card* = muscle, *itis* = inflammation or infection) that typically is caused by a previous viral infection.

- ✔ **Cardiomyopathy:** Cardiomyopathy is the name used for diseases of the heart muscle. Cardiomyopathies are characterized by whether they

  - Enlarge and weaken the heart muscle

  - Thicken and stiffen the heart muscle

  - Stiffen the heart muscle without thickening it

  I discuss cardiomyopathies in detail in Chapter 9.

Overloading the pump

As a pump, the heart may be compromised whenever it becomes inundated by:

- ✔ **Volume overloads:** The heart experiences a volume overload when it's asked to pump too much blood. These overloads typically result from leaking heart valves, which, in turn, cause torrential volumes of blood to leak back into the heart. This condition can overwhelm the heart, producing heart failure.

- ✔ **Pressure overloads:** The heart experiences a pressure overload when it's asked to pump against opposing pressures that it cannot adequately pump against. These overloads can occur either when a heart valve is narrowed *(stenosed)* or when the blood vessels have an increased resistance, such as occurs with hypertension.

Decreasing the heart's ability to fill adequately

The heart's pumping ability also is compromised when it can't take in adequate amounts of blood to pump out. Inadequate filling can occur when:

✔ Valves leading into the heart become narrowed

✔ The sac around the heart (the *pericardium*) becomes scarred and con-stricts the heart *(constrictive pericarditis)* or fills with fluid *(cardiac tamponade)* and presses down on the heart

✔ The heart muscle itself becomes so damaged that it becomes stiff and cannot relax enough to fill

Stressing caused by underlying conditions

A variety of underlying noncardiac illnesses and conditions also can cause a heart that is functioning marginally well to become stressed, tipping it over into heart failure. Such conditions include

✔ An overactive thyroid gland

✔ A systemic infection (a viral or bacterial infection that affects your whole body)

✔ A blood clot migrating to the lungs

✔ A low blood count

✔ Obstructive sleep apnea

✔ Alcohol abuse

✔ Any condition that increases the demands on the heart or decreases its ability to perform to the point that it fails as a pump

Recognizing the Symptoms of Heart Failure

Because heart failure produces a lack of blood flow to vital organs (including the heart) and muscles, the typical symptoms of heart failure are shortness of breath, fatigue, edema, and coughing.

Experiencing shortness of breath

Because the degree to which the heart's pumping ability has been compromised affects how short of breath you are, this symptom is classified on a scale of 1 to 4, ranging from shortness of breath only with vigorous exertion in Grade 1 to shortness of breath even while at rest in Grade 4. Doctors further divide the symptoms of shortness of breath into three categories that indicate when and where the shortness of breath occurs. (In typical medical fashion, each of these has a Latin name.)

- ✔ **Dyspnea,** which simply means shortness of breath, is the most prevalent and earliest symptom of heart failure. Dyspnea usually progresses so slowly that you subtly begin restricting activities to avoid the unpleasant sensation.

- ✔ **Orthopnea** is the inability to breathe comfortably while lying flat. Individuals with heart failure, particularly as it progresses, find they breathe more comfortably when the upper part of the body is elevated (on pillows or sitting).

- ✔ **Paroxysmal nocturnal dyspnea (PND)** is somewhat similar to orthopnea but describes transient episodes of severe shortness of breath that typically occur at night when you're lying down but may not be relieved merely by sitting upright.

Experiencing fatigue

Fatigue is a typical symptom of congestive heart failure. Inadequate blood flow to the muscles and other tissues causes fatigue, which makes accomplishing any level of significant exertion, or even the activities of daily living, difficult.

Recognizing mimics: Symptoms of heart failure that aren't

Even if it looks like a duck and walks like a duck, it may be a bear in disguise. The same is true in medicine: Some conditions have symptoms that mimic heart failure but stem from another ailment entirely. Shortness of breath or edema, for instance, may indicate a different problem. Typically, the conditions that cause shortness of breath are conditions of the lung, such as chronic obstructive pulmonary disease (COPD), asthma, or pulmonary infections. Conditions that cause edema include problems with either the liver or kidneys or problems with the veins. In each of these instances, a shrewd physician who takes a good history, performs a good physical examination, and judiciously orders the proper tests can distinguish between cardiac causes of shortness of breath and edema versus other conditions that may mimic congestive heart failure.

Experiencing edema and coughing

When the heart fails to pump adequately, fluid can accumulate in the feet, ankles, legs, and sometimes the abdomen, causing the swelling called edema. Fluid also can accumulate in the lungs, producing the congestion that gives congestive heart failure its name. For some individuals, lung congestion may result in persistent coughing or in wheezy or raspy breathing.

Diagnosing Heart Failure

Heart failure is diagnosed through a combination of a careful medical history, a thorough physical examination, and a number of cardiac tests. (For more details about each, check out Chapters 10 and 11.)

✔ **Medical history:** A history of any of the pulmonary symptoms (such as those described in the sidebar "Recognizing mimics: Symptoms of heart failure that aren't"), coupled with a history of heart disease, and/or a recent illness that may have tripped a previously overcompensated heart into heart failure, all point to a diagnosis of heart failure.

✔ **Physical examination:** During a physical examination, your physician may observe some of the more common signs.

- An extra heart sound (detected with the stethoscope — also called a *gallop*).

- Fluid in the lungs, which also can be detected with the stethoscope.

- An abnormal motion of the heart that indicates to the physician's touch that your heart is increased in size or is going through an abnormal contraction pattern.

- Abnormal pressures in the neck veins, which may be indicated by blood pressure measurements taken in both arms and sounds, *bruits,* that can be heard by stethoscope.

- *Pitting edema,* or fluid accumulation in the legs. When the physician presses down on the ankle, the impression left by the finger persists.

✔ **Laboratory tests:** Although no specific laboratory test for congestive heart failure exists, the following tests are useful.

- A complete blood chemical analysis and blood count indicates any abnormalities in liver function, in kidney function, and in electrolytes (indicators of fluid retention).

- An electrocardiogram often shows abnormalities of underlying heart disease that may have led to the heart failure.

- A chest X-ray shows accumulation of fluid in the lungs.

- Advanced cardiac tests, such as an echocardiogram and a nuclear test, indicate whether the heart is enlarged, show the condition of the valves, and provide an estimate of the ejection fraction. If the ejection fraction is 40 percent or less, the diagnosis of heart failure is highly likely.

- Heart catheterization and angiography occasionally are helpful in diagnosing heart failure because they enable the physician to measure pressures throughout the heart and lungs, which helps diagnose the type of heart failure. Looking at the coronary arteries also helps physicians decide whether heart failure is related to CAD.

Treating Heart Failure

Treatments for heart failure generally attempt to counteract the negative effects of the heart's own compensatory mechanisms, such as retaining fluids, or to strengthen the pumping ability of a weakened or damaged heart directly. These treatments range from lifestyle modifications to a variety of medicines and procedures.

Some of the treatment programs that you can undergo or that your doctor will institute to help treat heart failure are described in the sections that follow.

Modifying your lifestyle

Modifying certain lifestyle practices, as your doctor may direct, can help treat congestive heart failure and enhance the comfort and quality of your life as you live with the condition. Here are some of the things you'll be expected to do:

- **Weigh yourself.** You should weigh yourself every morning at the same time, typically after you've used the toilet but before you've eaten breakfast. Typically, physicians recommend that if you rapidly gain more than two pounds, you should contact your physician, because the weight gain may mean that your body is retaining fluid. If it is, you may require an adjustment in your medication.

- **Restrict sodium.** Because sodium causes your body to retain fluids, try to restrict your sodium intake. If you have heart failure, even a small increase in your sodium level can tip you over into a very serious bout of lung congestion.

✔ **Limit fluids and alcohol.** Alcohol consumption further depresses the pumping ability of the heart, and increased fluids can raise the fluid buildup in the lungs and the rest of the body. Heavy, long-term consumption of alcohol is a factor that can contribute to the development of heart failure.

✔ **Perform light or moderate exercise.** At one time, exercise wasn't recommended for people with heart failure. However, recent studies show that moderate exercise can help the heart pump more efficiently and other muscles work more efficiently. More efficient pumping and working reduces demands on the heart. Of course, if you experience heart failure, you won't be training for a marathon or triathlon — easy does it. Very carefully, too.

Before undertaking any exercise program, you absolutely must talk to your doctor about the amount and best type of exercise for you and the warning signs of overexercising.

✔ **Quit smoking.** If you smoke, quit. Your physician will urge you to make quitting your first priority. Smoking not only contributes to the underlying causes of heart failure but also has a direct effect on heart rate and blood pressure. (See Chapter 23 to find strategies for quitting smoking.)

Treating heart failure with medications

A variety of medicines, including several newly developed types, are useful in treating heart failure. Not all of these drugs are right for all patients, and combinations of drugs often are used to address individual situations. Here are some of the medicines that your physician may use.

✔ **Diuretics:** Often called *fluid pills* or *water pills* by the people who take them, diuretics help reduce the amount of fluid in the body and are useful in individuals who are experiencing heart failure and fluid retention. As I discuss in Chapter 13, diuretics also are useful in treating hypertension.

✔ **Digitalis:** Digitalis (or digoxin) helps the heart contract more vigorously. Digitalis was one of the first medicines to be used for treating heart failure. It initially was made from the foxglove plant — Latin name *digitalis*. (Deposit that in your trivia bank!) Digitalis continues to be one of the best medicines for stimulating the heart to pump more effectively and for reducing the symptoms of heart failure.

✔ **Angiotensin converting enzyme inhibitors (ACE inhibitors):** Although originally developed for treating high blood pressure, ACE inhibitors can reduce the work of the heart by decreasing the amount of pressure in blood vessels against which the heart must pump. Studies indicate this effect may slow losses in the heart's pumping ability and improve the quality of life and survival in people with heart failure.

Although these drugs have become an important part of the standard treatment of heart failure, several studies now show that many physicians underuse them. Feel free to ask your physician more about them.

✔ **Angiotensin II receptor blockers:** Your physician may choose to use these drugs in place of or, in some cases, in conjunction with ACE inhibitors. Research also shows that they may be useful for individuals who cannot take ACE inhibitors or beta blockers (see next item).

✔ **Beta blockers:** Because beta blockers (another drug developed to treat hypertension) slow the heart's contraction rate, thus reducing its pumping action, beta blockers for a long time were not considered appropriate for individuals with heart failure. Recent studies, however, suggest that certain beta blockers may actually be valuable to some patients with heart failure, probably because they reduce the likelihood that these patients will suffer significant heart rhythm problems.

✔ **Inotropes:** Inotropes are powerful medicines that make the heart contract more powerfully and must be delivered intravenously. Treatment with these drugs is almost always started in the hospital and typically is used only for carefully selected patients who have end-stage heart failure.

✔ **Aldosterone blockers:** These medicines block a hormone that causes the heart to retain fluid in heart failure. Recent studies show that using such drugs for heart-failure patients may significantly improves outcomes.

Treating heart failure with surgery

If medicines no longer are effective as you progressively slip into further heart failure, surgical techniques may be used to help you out. Several different surgical options are available.

✔ **Inserting a mechanical device to assist the heart:** In some cases, a mechanical pump called a *left ventricular assist device* (LVAD) may be sewn into the pumping chamber to assist a weakened heart. LVADs typically are reserved for use only as transitional devices in place for days or weeks when a patient is waiting for cardiac transplant. However, designs are being refined, and these devices are becoming available for long-term treatment.

✔ **Heart transplants:** The treatment of last resort for certain very severe, life-threatening cases of heart failure is a cardiac transplant. Replacing the entire heart in appropriate candidates has proven highly effective. A heart transplant can be lifesaving treatment for advanced heart failure. However, donor hearts are scarce, and other concerns, including organ rejection, limit the use of this option. Candidates for heart transplants are usually younger than 65 and have healthy vital organs (other than the heart) and no other life-threatening conditions or diseases.

✔ **Procedures to assist the heart muscle or shrink the size of the heart:** Such procedures still are considered experimental and used only in very severe cases of heart failure, and, even then, only by some surgeons who are particularly skilled in their application. None of these procedures is approved for wide use, but several areas of active research appear to hold promise.

- **Cellular cardiomyoplasty:** This procedure transplants cells that can stimulate the regeneration of muscle tissue (often skeletal muscle cells or bone marrow stem cells) within damaged cardiac muscle. The goal is improving the ability of damaged ventricular muscle to pump.

- **Dynamic cardiomyoplasty:** This procedure uses surgery to assist the heart or reduce the size of the ventricle. In one form of this procedure, a muscle from the back is partially rerouted, attached to the heart and electrically stimulated to beat to assist the heart; however, long-term muscle fatigue has proven to be a problem with this procedure. In another form of this procedure, left ventricular reduction (also known as the *Batista procedure*), a triangular section of left-ventricle muscle tissue is removed from an enlarged, weakened heart to reduce the size of the pumping chamber and increase its effectiveness.

- **Passive cardiomyoplasty:** This procedure uses *passive containment* — sometimes called a *heart jacket* — to wrap and support the heart muscle in a synthetic, elastic fabric. This passive support in some patients appears to increase heart function and even encourage heart muscle remodeling toward a more normal size. The reasons this change occurs are as yet unclear.

Working with Your Doctor to Fight Heart Failure

Because therapy for heart failure requires a great deal of precision and consistency, working carefully and closely with your physicians can help them maximize the effectiveness of any treatment. Here are some steps you can take to help control your heart failure:

✔ See your physician regularly, and don't be afraid to ask questions.

✔ Closely follow your physician's instructions.

✔ Take medication consistently and according to instructions.

✔ Follow recommended lifestyle practices.

✔ Immediately report to your physician any change in your condition, such as increased weight, shortness of breath, or swollen feet.

Chapter 8

Clotting and Bleeding in the Brain: Stroke

Stroke is common in the United States — in fact, it's the third leading cause of death in the U.S. behind heart disease and cancer. A stroke is also called a cerebral vascular accident (CVA) or, with increasing frequency these days, a brain attack. Regardless of how you refer to them, *strokes* are a type of cardiovascular disease, but because they primarily affect the brain, physicians and medical literature typically treat stroke as a separate condition.

Check out the following stroke statistics:

✔ Because of new treatments, many more people now survive strokes than did in the past. In fact, about 4.7 million American stroke survivors are alive today.

✔ Stroke affects men and women equally; however, women have about 40,000 more strokes per year than men because the average life expectancy for women is longer than for men. Before age 65, men have more strokes overall, but after age 65, women have more strokes than men. The elderly in general have higher stroke rates.

✔ For African Americans younger than 75, the risk of experiencing a stroke is two to four times higher than for European Americans, depending upon their respective ages.

✔ Although it's third on the list of causes of death, stroke takes center stage as the leading cause of serious long-term disability in the U.S. and is responsible for more than half of all hospitalizations for neurological disease.

Defining a Stroke

A stroke occurs when a blood clot or bleeding suddenly interrupts the flow of blood to an area of the brain. When deprived of blood, brain cells lose their ability to function and, if deprived for too long, die. Because brain cells and groups of brain cells have highly specialized functions, the location of stroke damage determines what loss of neurological and bodily function occurs as a result of stroke. Impairment may be temporary or permanent.

Understanding the types of stroke

Strokes are categorized in two basic ways: ischemic stroke and hemorrhagic stroke. The causes and results of stroke depend on how and where the stroke occurs.

Ischemic stroke

An ischemic stroke occurs when a blood clot or other particle blocks a blood vessel in the brain and cuts off the blood supply to the portion of the brain supplied by that vessel. Without adequate oxygen, that portion of the brain suffers damage or even dies, resulting in such typical stroke symptoms as paralysis or problems with speech, vision, or comprehension, depending on which portion of the brain is damaged. This type of stroke is called an *ischemic stroke* because it's caused by *ischemia,* the medical term for lack of blood flow. About 70 percent to 80 percent of all strokes are ischemic, and they occur in two basic forms.

- ✔ **Cerebral thrombosis:** This form of stroke results from progressive narrowing of arteries in the brain or sometimes in the carotid arteries in the neck. So what's the difference between a thrombosis and an embolism, the other type of ischemic stroke? In a thrombosis, plaque (there's that cholesterol again) that narrows the artery and any clot *(thrombus)* that forms on it don't move, meaning the typical underlying causes for this type of blockage are atherosclerosis and high blood pressure. Before having a major stroke, many people experience a temporary lack of blood flow to the brain that's called a *transient ischemic attack* (TIA), which actually is a small stroke in which the effects (such as those listed in the section "Recognizing the symptoms of a stroke" later in this chapter) usually last for only a few minutes or hours.

  Never ignore possible TIA symptoms; treat them as a serious warning and consult your physician.

- ✔ **Cerebral embolism:** This form of stroke occurs when a blood clot, or *embolus,* travels from somewhere else in the body to the brain. When the blood clot lodges in a vessel in the brain, it cuts off blood flow to the portion of the brain supplied by that vessel. Blood clots that cause strokes may form in and travel from a number of different locations in the body, including:

- Major arteries in the neck that supply the brain (the carotid arteries). This is why your doctor often listens with a stethoscope over your neck to hear whether any narrowing of one of these arteries has occurred. The narrowing of the artery leads to turbulence that the doctor can hear.

- The heart — particularly in people with atrial fibrillation. In this case, when the upper chambers, or atria, fibrillate instead of contracting normally, blood clots can form in the blood and travel directly from the left atrium to the brain.

Hemorrhagic stroke

A hemorrhagic stroke occurs when a blood vessel in or on the brain bursts and bleeds into the brain or into the space between the brain and skull. This type of stroke is called a hemorrhagic stroke because it's caused by a *hemorrhage* (in Greek, *hemo* means "blood" and *rhage* means "to break"). The brain is very sensitive to bleeding and pressure, which damage brain tissue, often permanently. Bleeding also irritates brain tissue, which swells to resist the expanding fluid. When contained, the blood forms a mass called a *hematoma;* it, too, exerts damaging pressure on brain tissue. Hemorrhagic strokes account for only about 20 percent of all strokes, but they usually are more severe and more often fatal than ischemic stroke. The two basic types of hemorrhagic stroke are

✔ **Cerebral hemorrhage or intracerebral hemorrhage (ICH):** This form of stroke occurs when an artery inside the brain ruptures and bleeds directly into the brain tissue surrounding the defective artery. Stress from chronic high blood pressure appears to play a primary role in damaging or weakening these small artery walls.

Other factors that may contribute to fragile vessels include

- Having a blood-clotting disorder

- Being on blood thinners or anticoagulants to treat heart disease or prevent ischemic stroke

- Having an accumulation of amyloid protein in the cerebral arteries

- Having an aneurysm

- Abusing cocaine

Occasionally, this type of stroke can occur during pregnancy because extra estrogen in the bloodstream can make blood vessels fragile. Sometimes cerebral hemorrhages occur as a complication of ischemic stroke.

✔ **Subarachnoid hemorrhage (SAH):** This form of stroke occurs when a blood vessel on the surface of the brain bursts and bleeds into the cavity between the skull and the brain. Blood filling this space pushes against the brain. In very severe bleeds, the pressure on the brain from blood pushing it against the skull can cause fatal damage. This kind of bleeding typically results from congenital abnormalities, such as *aneurysms,* which are weak spots on artery walls that can balloon out, or *arteriovenous malformations* (AVM), in which a brain artery attaches directly to a vein, bypassing any capillaries. A head injury also may cause this type of bleeding.

Recognizing the symptoms of a stroke

Stroke always is a medical emergency, and yet many people have difficulty recognizing the symptoms of stroke when they occur. Why? Well, for one thing, individual strokes may affect many different parts of the brain, so symptoms can vary widely from one stroke patient to the next. For another, although experts agree on a group of warning-sign symptoms, one or more of which typically are associated with stroke, many older people are among the most vulnerable to stroke and are unaware of these signs. Even if you're not at risk of stroke, you may nevertheless observe a loved one, co-worker, or neighbor experiencing symptoms of a possible stroke. Everyone needs to be keenly aware of and heed the warning signs of stroke.

Calling for medical help at the first sign of stroke offers the best opportunity for diagnosing and treating it within the first few hours of onset.

If you experience or see someone else experiencing one or more of the following symptoms, the National Institute of Neurological Disorders and Stroke and the Brain Attack Coalition strongly urge you to call 911 right away!

- ✔ Sudden numbness or weakness of the face, arm, or leg, especially on one side of the body
- ✔ Sudden confusion or trouble speaking or understanding speech
- ✔ Sudden trouble seeing in one or both eyes
- ✔ Sudden trouble walking, dizziness, or loss of balance or coordination
- ✔ Sudden severe headache with no known cause

Treatment can be more effective if it's given immediately. Every minute counts!

Reviewing risk factors for stroke

As is true of coronary artery disease (CAD), a number of factors can increase your risk of having a stroke. Some factors, such as age and heredity, are out of your hands, but you can do much to control risk factors that are related to lifestyle choices.

Risk factors you can't change

Although you can't change the risk factors in the following list, understanding them may increase your awareness and help you make better choices about the risk factors you can control.

- ✔ **Age:** Although many people younger than 65 have strokes, the risk of stroke doubles with each decade after age 55.

- ✔ **Heredity and family history:** Your risk of having a stroke is higher if a parent, grandparent, or sibling has had a stroke. Certain inherited genetic traits, such as blood-clotting disorders, and family lifestyle patterns likely contribute to this elevated risk.

- ✔ **Gender:** Although men and women have about the same overall risk of having a stroke, women are more likely to die from stroke. Taking birth control pills also slightly increases the risk of stroke particularly when combined with other risk factors like smoking or high blood pressure.

- ✔ **Previous stroke:** Having had one stroke greatly increases your risk of having another stroke. For this reason, preventing recurrent stroke is an important goal in the long-term health-care plan for stroke survivors.

Risk factors you can control

Controlling one or more of these risk factors can significantly lower your risk of stroke. Having one of these risk factors will raise your risk of stroke. Having a cluster or two or three factors, which is a fairly common circumstance, dramatically raises your risk of stroke.

- ✔ **High blood pressure:** Having high blood pressure is perhaps the greatest risk factor for stroke. In fact, the higher your blood pressure, the greater the risk. Controlling blood pressure within normal ranges can lower this risk.

- ✔ **Smoking:** Because smoking damages the cardiovascular system all over the body, and not just in the heart, it damages vessels in the brain and the carotid arteries leading to the brain and contributes to the narrowing of these vessels.

- ✔ **Heart disease:** People with heart disease and people who've had heart attacks are at higher risk of stroke. Having atrial fibrillation is a particularly significant risk factor because embolitic clots often form during atrial fibrillation.

- ✔ **Diabetes:** Not only is having diabetes an independent risk factor for stroke, but people with diabetes often have high blood pressure, high cholesterol, and weight problems, all of which are additional factors that increase stroke risk.

- ✔ **Substance abuse:** Binge drinking or even drinking beyond recommended moderate levels (no more than one drink daily for women and two for men) raises the risk of stroke. Intravenous drug abuse can lead to cerebral embolisms; cocaine abuse also has been linked to stroke.

Five tips for lowering your risk of stroke

Prevention is the most important treatment against stroke. The development of more effective treatment of hypertension during the last 20 years, for example, has lowered the prevalence of stroke in the U.S. — and that's a major breakthrough. Following these lifestyle practices will help you lower your risk of stroke:

✔ Treating high blood pressure

✔ Quitting smoking

✔ Managing heart disease

✔ Controlling diabetes

✔ Seeking help for transient ischemic attacks (TIAs)

Diagnosing and Treating Stroke in the ER

When someone who's experiencing stroke symptoms arrives in the hospital emergency room, the medical-care team moves immediately to determine whether that person is experiencing a stroke or some other neurological illness. The medical team takes a number of almost simultaneous steps to diagnose and evaluate the type and severity of the stroke by:

✔ Asking questions to assess when symptoms began and the patient's alertness, symptoms, and degree of impairment. Most people experiencing a stroke are conscious, but if the patient is unable able to respond, the medical team usually seeks this information from accompanying family members or associates.

✔ Establishing whether the patient is able to breathe easily.

✔ Checking vital signs including blood pressure, heart function (including possible arrhythmia), body temperature, and blood oxygen and glucose (sugar) levels.

Another initial step in diagnosing and evaluating a stroke victim is determining whether the stroke is ischemic or hemorrhagic. Making this determination is critically important because these forms of brain attacks require very different treatment. The variety of tests that physicians use in making this determination include

✔ Asking questions about the onset, symptoms, impairments, and basic patient history that yield vital clues to the type of stroke that has occurred.

✔ Examining the patient to assess the nature and extent of impairments, thus providing additional clinical indicators of the type of stroke.

✔ Performing a CT scan as quickly as possible to provide images that indicate whether the stroke involves bleeding into the brain (hemorrhagic) or blocked blood flow (ischemic). These images also provide information about the size and area of the brain affected by the stroke and the blood vessels involved in the stroke.

• If the stroke is ischemic, the medical team evaluates whether to administer clot-busting medications, such as *tPA (tissue plasminogen activator)*. In carefully selected cases, such medications may improve or restore blood flow to the stroke-damaged areas of the brain or adjacent tissues, thus lessening the serious problems that can result from stroke. However, clot-busting therapy is not appropriate for all ischemic strokes. In addition, it is effective only when administered within three hours of the onset of stroke symptoms.

Unfortunately, the American Stroke Association estimates that only 3 percent to 5 percent of people who experience a stroke ever arrive at the hospital within this three-hour window. The potential for using this therapy is an important reason for noting when symptoms begin.

• If the stroke is hemorrhagic, the medical-care team first determines the cause of the bleeding, such as aneurysm or AVM, and then evaluates whether emergency surgery to repair the rupture is appropriate.

✔ As the stroke patient is stabilized, the medical-care team carries out additional diagnostic studies, screening for complications and establishing the extent of the stroke. The timing of these tests depends on the condition of the patient.

Managing Stroke in the Hospital

After confirming a diagnosis of stroke and stabilizing the patient, the ER doctor admits the patient into the hospital, usually into an intensive care unit (ICU). There the medical-care team observes the patient closely and manages care to assist in recovery and prevent complications whenever possible. Typically the first 24 to 48 hours after a stroke are the most critical. The medical management of a stroke patient's case usually involves several elements:

✔ **Monitoring critical signs that can signal potential complications.** Depending on the patient, these vital signs may include blood pressure, *intracranial pressure* (pressure inside the skull), breathing, and heart performance.

✔ **Performing additional diagnostic tests to determine the location, extent of the tissue affected, and possible causes of the stroke.**

Such tests may include

- CT scans or multimodal magnetic resonance imaging (MRI) to show what the injured brain looks like.

- Electroencephalograms (EEGs) to measure the brain's electrical activity.

- Evoked response tests to assess the brain's sensory functions, such as vision, touch, and hearing.

- Perfusion tests, such as various ultrasound tests, PET scan, or angiograms, that assess blood flow to the brain.

- Various cardiac tests to determine whether underlying heart disease played a role in the stroke. (See Chapter 11 for more about most of these diagnostic tests.)

✔ **Providing appropriate drug therapy and medical treatment to manage potential complications and improve recovery.**

Depending on the patient, such treatments may include

- Using antiplatelet agents (such as aspirin) and/or anticoagulants to prevent clotting

- Preventing seizures

- Reducing intracranial pressure

- Enhancing blood flow to the brain

- Controlling extremely high blood pressure

✔ **Performing surgical procedures that will improve the chances for recovery.**

Depending on the type of stroke, such procedures include

- Relieving intracranial pressure

- Repairing a ruptured aneurysm or AVM with a clip or endovascular coil that seals off the damaged portion of the vessel

- Removing a hematoma that's placing too much pressure on the brain

- Performing a carotid endarterectomy, which removes severe blockages

✔ **Planning for long-term rehabilitation to improve brain function and recovery of abilities and making the transition to the appropriate programs and services.**

Before the stroke survivor is discharged from the hospital, the medical-care team typically determines what specific rehabilitation services the patient needs and places the patient and family in contact with these services.

Recovering from Stroke

The leading cause of serious disability for American adults is stroke. No contest. However, after stroke damages part of the brain, the appropriate rehabilitation therapy can help stroke survivors regain better function and, in many cases, recover normal function entirely. Making full use of rehabilitation services, such as physical therapy, occupational therapy, speech therapy, and psychological therapy help patients regain as much functional ability as possible. The good news is that the brain is wonderfully *plastic* — meaning it has the ability to learn and change, with healthy parts taking over for injured parts. As a consequence, some stroke patients are able to regain full or satisfactory function. Making appropriate modifications to the home also helps many stroke survivors live well and safely even if they experience some limitations.

Your physician and the medical-care team at the hospital typically work with you and your family to plan appropriate rehabilitation services after you suffer a stroke. If you don't think you have adequate information, don't be shy about asking questions. For a quick, complete overview, I recommend a handy booklet, "Recovering After a Stroke: A Patient and Family Guide." It's Consumer Guide 16 from the U.S. Agency for Healthcare Research and Quality. You can order it by calling 800-358-9295 or download it online from the Internet Stroke Center at `www.strokecenter.org/pat/ras_toc.htm`.

Finding More Information about Stroke

The following organizations provide a wealth of information about stroke and resources for stroke patients and their families:

- **The National Institute of Neurological Disorders and Stroke** provides plenty of useful information on its Web site (`www.ninds.nih.gov`). You may also reach its public information office at the following address: **NIH Neurological Institute,** P.O. Box 5801, Bethesda, MD 20892; phone 800-352-9424.

- **The Internet Stroke Center,** a project of the University of Washington School of Medicine in St. Louis, provides a wide range of information on stroke. It also offers links to other resources. Web site: `www.strokecenter.org`.

- **The American Stroke Association,** a division of the American Heart Association, provides a variety of information, including news of local events that the association sponsors across the country. It publishes *Stroke Connection,* a free magazine for stroke survivors and their families. The Heart and Stroke Encyclopedia A to Z Guide provides information on a wide range of topics. Phone: 888-478-7653; Web site: `www.strokeassociation.org`.

✔ **The National Stroke Association** provides education, information, research, and referrals, and sponsors nationwide chapters and support groups. Phone: 800-787-6537; Web site: www.stroke.org.

✔ **The National Rehabilitation Information Center** provides excellent access to online databases and resources. Phone: 800-346-2742; Web site: www.naric.com.

Other helpful sites include the National Heart, Lung, and Blood Institute (www.nhlbi.nih.gov), the Mayo Clinic (www.mayohealth.org), and Johns Hopkins Health Information (www.intelihealth.com).

Chapter 9

Identifying Other Cardiac Conditions

*I*n this chapter, I look at a variety of conditions in which the heart plays a major role — but usually not the only role. In a sense, this chapter is a kind of grab bag of heart problems. Although each condition covered in this chapter affects fewer Americans than coronary artery disease and its major risk factors, these conditions are hardly minor — particularly when you or a family member has one. Plus, most of these conditions also have links to coronary heart disease. So, buckle your seat belts for a quick tour of other important cardiac conditions. I describe each condition, hit the highlights of treatment, and tell you where you can find more information if you need it.

Understanding Peripheral Vascular Disease

When disease narrows the arteries of the heart, it's called *coronary artery disease* (CAD). When that same disease process affects other arteries, particularly in the arms and legs, it's called *peripheral vascular disease* (PVD) or *peripheral artery disease* (PAD). And don't think peripheral means unimportant.

Identifying the causes of peripheral vascular disease

The narrowing of arteries in the body's extremities happens the same way as it does in the coronary arteries. Fatty plaques composed of cholesterol, other lipids, and proteins build up on the artery walls to produce atherosclerosis. This condition affects about 12 percent of people ages 65 to 70 and 20 percent of those older than 70, or a total of about 10 million Americans. PVD is particularly common in cigarette smokers, and it's more common in men than in women. The most common arteries involved are those of the legs.

Although many people with peripheral vascular disease never experience symptoms, the most common symptom is pain in the leg muscles during exertion such as fast walking or climbing a hill or stairs. In medicine, this leg discomfort is called *claudication*. This discomfort or pain usually goes away when you're at rest *(intermittent claudication)*, but if the arteries are totally or nearly blocked, the pain can persist even while you're resting. Severe blockage can lead to severe complications, such as leg ulcers and, rarely, tissue death requiring amputation. Having PVD also puts you at higher risk of heart attack and stroke.

Diagnosing peripheral vascular disease

Experiencing recurring pain in your legs like what I describe above signals the need to see your physician. When checking for the possibility of PVD, your doctor asks a number of questions about your symptoms and performs a simple test called an *ankle brachial index* (ABI). Performing an ABI consists of taking your blood pressure in both ankles (legs) and both arms and determining from those readings a specific ratio that gives your doctor a good indication of whether your peripheral arteries are narrowing. When that's what your doctor finds, he or she may order additional tests to determine the extent of blockage present. Typical tests include MRI angiography, X-ray angiography, and Doppler ultrasound (see Chapter 13).

Treating peripheral vascular disease

A number of treatments are available to relieve the lack of blood flow to the legs caused by peripheral vascular disease.

✔ **Progressively (and slowly) increasing physical activity:** Gradually increasing your physical activity usually is the first recommendation for patients with intermittent pain. Directed by your physician, a daily program of moderate and slowly progressive exercise can improve physical fitness and help develop *collateral circulation,* alternate circulation through smaller blood vessels. Your doctor may also prescribe medications to improve circulation and lower your chances for developing blood clots. These medications include antiplatelet and anticoagulant therapies. Typically more than 70 percent of patients using these treatment regimens improve or maintain their condition.

Because circulation often is poor in the lower leg, taking good care of your feet is important. That includes avoiding tight socks and injury. Poor circulation in the feet makes even small injuries such as blisters potentially dangerous because the injury is slow to heal and any infection is difficult to treat. If you have peripheral vascular disease, be sure you understand and religiously carry out your doctor's instructions for proper foot care.

✔ **Modifying lifestyle behaviors to lower your risk of developing atherosclerosis:** Taking this step helps slow or even stop the process of narrowing in the peripheral arteries. Quitting smoking is a particularly helpful modification.

✔ **Restoring blood flow through nonsurgical and surgical treatments:** When the narrowing of your arteries is severe, these treatments can include balloon angioplasty (usually using stents), a technique similar to the procedure used to open coronary arteries (see Chapter 13). However, in this case, the balloon-tipped catheter is threaded into the narrowed artery of the leg and expanded to open up the artery and allow more blood flow to occur. In selected cases, your physician may recommend bypass graft surgery to bypass the blockages and restore blood flow.

Understanding Valvular Heart Disease

As I discuss in Chapter 2, the four heart valves serve as traffic cops of the heart, directing blood flow in the proper direction and preventing it from improperly backing up.

As long as these valves open fully and shut tightly, all is well. But if any disease or injury causes valve leakage *(regurgitation)* or narrowing *(stenosis),* major problems can result. Significant valve leakage can overload the heart because extra blood flowing back into the heart requires an extrastrong beat to eject it. A narrowed valve can cause the heart to thicken because it is being asked to pump against a much higher pressure.

Identifying common valve malfunctions and their causes

Regurgitation and stenosis are the two most common valve malfunctions, or conditions that cause malfunctions. Although either condition can affect any or all valves, the mitral and aortic valves in the left heart, the main pumping chamber, are the ones usually affected. Both conditions can, and often do, exist simultaneously in either the same valve or different valves. A number of different conditions cause valves to leak or narrow, including:

- ✔ Congenital valvular problems (a condition you're born with).

- ✔ Damage to valve structures, such as when the structures that anchor the flaps of the mitral valve break.

- ✔ Progressive problems, including those that may result from the aging process, such as calcification, or those that result from an infection, such as rheumatic fever or endocarditis. If the problem becomes too severe, it may require open-heart surgery and valve replacement.

A couple of specific conditions need an extra word:

- ✔ **Mitral valve prolapse:** This condition is a ballooning backward of the mitral valve when the heart contracts. During physical examination, it produces a murmur and "click" heard through the stethoscope. This condition is particularly common in adolescents and young adults, especially women. Six percent to 10 percent of young women have mitral valve prolapse. (For reasons that are totally unclear, thin, young women are most often affected.)

    In any event, knowing whether you have mitral valve prolapse is important, because this condition makes you more susceptible to infections of the heart valve. Such infections can damage the valve enough to require surgical replacement.

- ✔ **Infectious endocarditis:** Heart valves can be infected with bacteria that have been introduced into the bloodstream in various ways. This condition is called *infectious endocarditis*. Although normal heart valves may contract endocarditis, it's much more common in hearts that have an underlying valve problem. Bacteria spilling into the bloodstream from dental work is a common cause of endocarditis. An infection elsewhere in the body may also cause bacteria to enter the bloodstream. Unfortunately, no symptoms specific to endocarditis enable you to identify it, but the possibility of contracting it is another reason to visit the doctor whenever you experience a persistent fever or other symptoms of infection such as night sweats, chills, or loss of appetite.

Although these infections of the heart valve can become very serious, they usually can be effectively treated with intravenous antibiotics lasting anywhere from two to six weeks. However, in some instances, the infection can become so destructive that one or more valves may need to be replaced.

The best advice: If you know that you have mitral valve prolapse with regurgitation (leakage) or any underlying valve abnormality, make sure that you take antibiotics, both prior to and after undergoing any medical procedure that might allow bacteria to enter the bloodstream — even if it's "only" a dental procedure or minor surgery. Ask your physician if you need to take antibiotics in these circumstances and which antibiotics are right for you.

Diagnosing valve problems

Because valve problems produce broad rather than specific symptoms, your physician will use your symptoms and a physical exam — in particular, a close listen to your heart with a stethoscope — when considering whether your problem may be valvular. The doctor may order further tests as necessary, including a chest X-ray and an echocardiogram, the latter of which provides images of your heart valves in action. Additionally, an MRI can produce a three-dimensional image of the valves and heart. (See Chapter 13 for more about these diagnostic tools.)

Treating valve problems

If a valve abnormality is not progressing rapidly or causing any serious problem, your physician may simply keep a close eye on it so that treatment can be initiated when and if it becomes necessary. Following a heart-healthy diet and lifestyle can also support valve health. Taking preventive antibiotics as needed when you have an underlying valve abnormality is a good idea.

Various nonsurgical and surgical techniques like the ones in the list that follows may be performed to correct valve problems.

- ✔ Balloon catheter procedures *(balloon valvuloplasty)* can be used in certain situations to widen a narrowed valve.

- ✔ Surgical modification and repair can be used to correct other valve problems.

✔ Valve replacement with either a pig's valve (porcine valve) or mechanical valve offers very effective treatment when a diseased valve cannot be repaired. Because blood clots may form on foreign surfaces of any mechanical valve, people who have these replacements must take anticoagulants for as long as they have the mechanical valve, usually the rest of their lives. Porcine valves rarely require anticoagulants, but they typically don't last as long as mechanical valves and must be replaced more often.

Understanding Diseases of the Aorta

Think of the aorta as the major superhighway leading out of the heart. For every organ in the body, including the heart, blood must first flow into and through the aorta before being efficiently distributed to all of the working tissues. (See Figure 9-1.)

A healthy aorta can take the pounding of being right next to the heart and the regular thrusts of large volumes of blood being ejected into it with each heart beat. However, various conditions can cause the aorta to malfunction. *Catastrophic* doesn't begin to describe what that means.

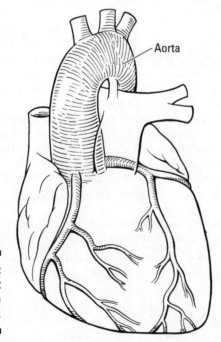

Aorta

Figure 9-1:
The heart
and the
aorta.

Identifying the causes of aorta problems

The most common problems of the aorta arise from the same disease process that affects the coronary arteries, mainly atherosclerosis.

When the aorta becomes hardened from atherosclerosis, it can leak or even break apart, a condition called an *aortic dissection.* Aortic dissection may also be triggered by high blood pressure, pregnancy (presumably because the aorta is weakened by the extra estrogen floating around the body), or in certain abnormalities of the connective tissue. One such connective tissue abnormality is a usually hereditary condition called Marfan's syndrome, which is characterized by elongated bones, looseness in the joints and fragmentation of connective fibers in the wall of the aorta — among other things. A number of professional athletes have actually died from aortic dissections caused by Marfan's.

Aneurysms, or weaknesses in the artery wall that cause it to balloon out, also occur in the aorta. Although these aneurysms can occur adjacent to the heart, they more commonly occur in the section of the aorta that travels down the middle of the body. In this latter case, the problem is called an *abdominal aortic aneurysm* (AAA).

Diagnosing aorta problems

Aortic problems rarely produce symptoms. An aortic dissection, for example, usually occurs suddenly without warning. Detecting an aortic aneurysm earlier is possible and more common. Your doctor often can feel an aortic aneurysm by placing his or her hands on the abdomen. Because developing aneurysms exhibit no symptoms, the potential for experiencing one is another reason for having regular thorough physical exams. After you're diagnosed with an aneurysm, it needs to be carefully examined, because as it continues to expand, an aneurysm can actually rupture, which results in a catastrophic outcome, usually death. Additional tests that are typically used to diagnose aorta problems are a basic chest X-ray, echocardiogram, MRI, abdominal ultrasound, and CT scan.

Treating aorta conditions

A leaking aorta is a medical emergency. A ruptured aorta is frequently fatal. An aorta that leaks or is in danger of rupturing requires surgery to replace the weakened section with a woven Dacron graft. This surgery needs to be performed by a highly skilled surgeon who is familiar with this delicate procedure, because the potential for problems with coronary arteries, in addition to the aorta, is very high.

Understanding Pericarditis

Normally the *pericardium,* the thin sac surrounding the heart, is lubricated with bodily fluids, enabling the heart to move freely as it contracts and relaxes. When the pericardium becomes inflamed or infected, a condition called *pericarditis,* it can threaten rather than protect the health of your heart.

Identifying the causes of pericarditis

A number of conditions can cause pericarditis, including bacterial or viral infections, inflammation, diseases of the connective tissue, and even cancer. In a sense, many of these conditions are a result of the pericardium serving as the last defense against invasion of the heart; however, when these conditions occur, they can cause the pericardium to malfunction. Your heart's ability to function can be impeded by fluid that builds up in the pericardial sac or fibrous tissue that infiltrates the pericardial sac after an infection.

Individuals with pericarditis often have chest discomfort when they breathe deeply or when they lie down. Pain when swallowing, coughing, and fever also can accompany pericarditis. A buildup of excess fluid also can occur between the pericardium and the heart, a condition called *pericardial effusion.*

Diagnosing pericarditis

Your symptoms are the first signs leading your physician to look for pericarditis. A stethoscope exam may reveal rubbing sounds typical of fluid around the heart. An echocardiogram is one of the best tests for confirming fluid buildup around the heart and the diagnosis of pericarditis. Your physician also may order other imaging studies like chest X-rays, CT scans, or MRIs (see Chapter 13).

Treating pericarditis

Treating pericarditis requires treating the underlying condition. If pericarditis is caused by a bacterial infection, antibiotics and draining the effusion away from the heart — through a needle *(pericardiocentesis)* or through surgery — are typical therapies for resolving the pericarditis. On rare occasions, the pericardium must be removed surgically, but you can get along well without it. Pericarditis often gets better with treatment using a nonsteroid anti-inflammatory drug (NSAID) such as ibuprofen.

Understanding Diseases of the Heart Muscle

As I discuss in Chapter 7, certain conditions called cardiomyopathies can actually harm the heart muscle. About 50,000 Americans suffer from a form of cardiomyopathy. And these conditions are the leading reason for heart transplants.

Identifying types and causes of cardiomyopathies

The term *cardiomyopathy* literally means "disease of the heart muscle" (*cardio* = heart; *myo* = muscle; *pathy* = disease), and doctors speak of *cardiomyopathies* because the term covers a number of conditions. These conditions typically are classified according to the three basic effects that they have on the heart muscle and its function. Each type of cardiomyopathy may have many different causes.

- ✔ **Congestive cardiomyopathy:** In this type, the heart becomes *dilated,* or enlarged, and heart muscle loses its ability to contract well. A virus often causes this type of damage, but other conditions that can also cause congestive cardiomyopathy include damage from chronic, excessive alcohol consumption. In many cases, the cause is *idiopathic,* or unidentified.

- ✔ **Hypertrophic cardiomyopathy:** In this type, the heart muscle thickens, or becomes *hypertrophied.* Although the heart continues to contract well, the thickening of the muscle makes the pumping chamber smaller and keeps the heart muscle from relaxing properly between contractions. Hypertrophic cardiomyopathy is an inherited condition in more than half of the cases. Heart valve disease and high blood pressure are risk factors that can lead to this condition.

- ✔ **Restrictive cardiomyopathy:** In this type, which is rare in the United States, abnormal tissue may be deposited or grow within the heart muscle itself, causing the muscle to become stiff. This problem can occur when radiation is administered to the chest (for example, to treat a tumor elsewhere in the chest) or in certain connective tissue diseases.

Diagnosing cardiomyopathies

The warning signs of possible cardiomyopathy are shortness of breath, bloating, fainting, and chest pain. If you experience these symptoms, your physician will perform or order tests to confirm or rule out cardiomyopathy. For example, a chest X-ray can show whether the heart is enlarged. An echocardiogram can reveal heart size and muscle damage. An electrocardiogram (ECG) also can provide information about the condition of the heart's pumping chambers. Various imaging tests such as echocardiogram, heart catheterization, and nuclear stress test, may provide information on the heart's pumping ability.

Treating cardiomyopathies

The therapy for cardiomyopathies depends on the underlying condition and the type of cardiomyopathy. If an infection causes it, treatment of the infection is very important. In addition, other medicinal and surgical treatments may be employed to help the heart contract properly. Because advanced cardiomyopathies generally lead to heart failure, you may find my discussion of the treatment for heart failure in Chapter 7 helpful. In most cases, the goal of the treatment regimen is reducing the symptoms and enhancing the heart's function because, in most cases, changes to the heart muscle cannot be reversed.

Understanding Pulmonary Embolism and Deep Vein Thrombosis (DVT)

A blood clot that travels into the lungs is called a *pulmonary embolus*. Unfortunately, more than a half million Americans experience episodes of blood clots entering their lungs every year, and about 200,000 of these people die as a result. In many cases the clot in the lung arises from *deep vein thrombosis* (DVT).

Identifying the causes of pulmonary embolism

Pulmonary embolism, a clot that travels to an artery in the lungs and blocks it, typically is the result of an underlying disease. For example, people with certain types of cancer may have blood that is particularly likely to clot and cause pulmonary blood clots to the lungs. Pulmonary embolisms also are a danger for people who experience a condition called *deep vein thrombosis,* where a clot forms in a vessel in the legs or pelvis, which can result from prolonged bed rest or inactivity. Other risk factors include certain medications (such as birth control pills) and inherited clotting disorders.

The two major sources of pulmonary embolisms are

✔ Blood clots that form in the pelvic veins and deep veins of the legs — DVT. These clots, by far the most common type, break loose and travel into the right side of the heart. They are then ejected into the lung circulation where they can block blood flow to a portion of the lung.

✔ Blood clots that in some instances can actually form in the right side of the heart itself, particularly in patients with atrial fibrillation.

Diagnosing pulmonary embolism

Because a pulmonary embolism can be life-threatening, diagnosing and treating the condition as quickly as possible is important. Shortness of breath, pain associated with breathing, and sudden onset of wheezing can be symptoms. Certainly any sudden or rapidly developing shortness of breath should send you right to the doctor or emergency room. Unfortunately, this condition produces no symptoms (or only vague symptoms) in many cases, particularly when circulating blood clots are very small. The most specific tests used to confirm pulmonary embolism are spiral CT scan and *nuclear V/Q scan,* which provides images of the blood flow *(perfusion)* to the lungs. Your physician or medical-care team typically uses a range of tests to rule out other conditions that may have symptoms similar to pulmonary embolism.

Treating pulmonary embolism

Anticoagulants (blood thinners) are the most common treatment for a blood clot to the lungs. This regimen often begins with intravenous drugs such as Heparin followed by three to six months of anticoagulation with medicines that are taken by mouth. When blood clots are particularly dangerous or recurrent, a mechanical filter may also be placed in the veins coming out of the legs to actually catch the blood clots before they reach the heart and lungs.

People who have had one episode of deep vein thrombosis or pulmonary embolism are at elevated risk for repeat episodes. If you're one of those people, your physician may recommend preventive treatments, including medications, lifestyle modifications, and wearing support hose.

Understanding Cor Pulmonale

I devote an entire chapter to heart failure (Chapter 7), which is caused by problems with the heart itself. When the right the right side of the heart fails because of conditions in the lungs (not the heart), it's called (in Latin, natch) *cor pulmonale* (*cor* = heart, *pulmonale* = lungs).

In cor pulmonale, disorders of the lungs, such as emphysema, cause pressures to rise in the blood circulation in the lungs. This pressure in turn causes the right side of the heart to fail in its job of pumping blood into the lungs.

Treating the underlying disorder is, by far, the most effective way to deal with cor pulmonale. Certainly, stopping cigarette smoking or other irritants to the lung is very important. In addition, individuals may benefit from blood-thinning medicines to prevent blood clots from traveling to the lungs. Occasionally, lung transplant surgery is required to correct underlying lung problems that cause the right side of the heart to fail.

Understanding Congenital Heart Disease

Congenital heart disease in adults is quite rare. Congenital heart disease in newborns complicates about 1percent of births. Treatment of various congenital abnormalities is in the domain of the pediatric cardiologist and the pediatric cardiac surgeon. When an adult patient is diagnosed with congenital heart disease, the defect probably escaped detection in childhood. Why? The defect may have been very subtle, misdiagnosed as a benign condition, or the result of inadequate medical attention. As treatment of congenital heart disease has progressed, however, more people with congenital heart disease are reaching adulthood. A team approach between pediatric and adult cardiologists benefits these patients as they grow from youth to adulthood.

More than 90 percent of adults with congenital heart disease have one of these five conditions.

- **Atrial septal defect (ASD):** An abnormal opening or hole in the septum between the two atria

- **Ventricular septal defect (VSD):** An abnormal opening or hole in the septum between the two ventricles

- **Pulmonic stenosis (PS):** A narrowing of the valve leading from the right side of the heart into the lungs

- **Patent ductus arteriosus (PDA):** An abnormal connection from the aorta to the pulmonary artery

- **Coarctation of the aorta (COARC):** A narrowing of the aorta occurring beyond the aortic valve

The treatment of congenital conditions typically requires surgical correction of the underlying defect. Atrial septal defects, however, may now be closed with less-invasive catheter-based therapies. Occasionally, medicines may be used, either as a transitional phase to support patients until they're ready for surgery, or as part of the overall therapy.

Understanding Cardiac Tumors

Like any other organ, the heart is susceptible to various tumor growths. Fortunately, these *cardiac tumors* are quite rare. Unfortunately, when the heart is involved with a tumor, it is three times more likely to be a metastatic tumor that has spread from another organ system than a tumor of the heart itself. Most tumors that metastasize to the heart are close anatomically. These include lung cancers, in particular, and cancers that travel in the bloodstream (breast cancer, melanoma, and leukemia). Major tumors of the heart muscle itself are quite rare.

When the tumor is metastatic, treatment of the underlying primary cancer usually is the best course of action. Tumors of the heart muscle itself are treated with chemotherapy, radiation, and/or occasionally surgery.

Understanding Cardiac Trauma

Just like any other organ in the body, the heart can be injured in various traumatic ways, including penetrating or nonpenetrating chest injuries. The most common type of cardiac trauma occurs in an automobile accident when the chest slams against the steering wheel (another good reason to wear your seat belt). In some instances, cardiac trauma may be overlooked because other types of trauma may be more obvious. Because the ribs and muscles inside the chest cavity strongly defend the heart, it is relatively well protected. However, serious cardiac trauma can be fatal.

If the heart actually is penetrated (in medicine this is called a *laceration*), blood can leak into the pericardium, rapidly causing death. Suspecting and then checking for cardiac trauma is important anytime an individual has been in a setting where it can occur, such as a motor-vehicle accident. Recognition and rapid diagnosis of the injury through techniques such as echocardiography may prove to be lifesaving.

Surgery typically is required whenever significant cardiac trauma occurs. When you're in an automobile accident in which your chest hits the steering wheel, physicians and patients alike need to be alert to the possibility that cardiac trauma has occurred.

Finding More Information

For additional information about these and other diseases of the heart, the Web site of the American Heart Association (www.americanheart.org) offers an easy-to-use reference guide, "Heart and Stroke Encyclopedia." Other helpful Web sites include the National Heart, Lung, and Blood Institute (www.nhlbi.nih.gov), the Mayo Clinic (www.mayohealth.org), and Johns Hopkins Health Information (www.intelihealth.com).

Part III
Finding Out Whether You Have Heart Disease

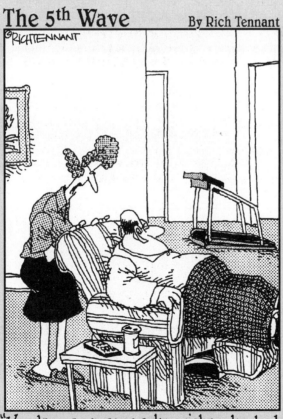

The 5th Wave   By Rich Tennant

"You know, anyone who wishes he had a remote control for his exercise equipment is missing the idea of exercise equipment."

In this part . . .

These chapters offer a quick but thorough guide to
the many techniques, tests, and procedures that your
primary-care physician and cardiologist may use in assessing your heart health and heart disease. I look first at the
importance of a regular physical exam and personal health
history and then detail exactly what's behind all those
letters (ECG, CT, MRI, PET) in the most common diagnostic
tests and procedures used in evaluating heart disease.
Finally, I share strategies and tips for building an effective
health-care partnership with your doctor.

Chapter 10

Taking the First Step: Going for a Checkup

*T*he health fair test showed my total cholesterol count is 250, should I do something about that? Does the chest pain I'm having indicate heart problems? If heart disease is the number-one health problem, do I already have heart disease?

Such scary questions occur to almost everyone sooner or later in life. The later, the better, most people hope. Your physicians hope so, too. That's why assessing your risk factors for heart disease over time — when you go in for regular checkups or even for an acute problem like the flu — is a priority for your physician. Continual assessment of your risks should be a priority for you and every member of your family. Remember that your health and well-being depend in large measure on the health and well-being of the old ticker.

Regardless of whether you're the picture of perfect health, you've already been diagnosed with heart disease, or you've experienced a cardiac event, you can work with your physician on evaluating your risk of various manifestations of heart disease, on the primary prevention of heart disease by controlling risk factors, and if you already have heart disease, on implementing secondary prevention of disease progression and additional cardiac events.

Tuning In to Your Heart and Health

Your primary-care physician may be keeping an eye on your heart health, but how often do you see him or her? Nobody knows your life, your usual habits and activities, and how you feel better than you do. You keep a watchful eye on your bank account, don't you? Just to make sure nothing goes awry? Tuning in to your heart's well-being is even more important.

Several simple steps can make you an active partner in maintaining your heart health at the highest levels and can help you take quick, positive action at the first sign of any trouble.

✔ **Schedule a regular checkup.** In the section "Going for a Checkup: The Medical History and Physical Examination" later in this chapter, I detail the diagnostic techniques your physician regularly uses to assess your current heart health and potential problems.

✔ **Know the risk factors for heart disease (see Chapter 3).** These include high blood pressure, elevated cholesterol, physical inactivity, obesity, smoking, and diabetes.

✔ **Follow the daily lifestyle practices that are good for your overall health and quality of life.** Practices that lower the risk factors for heart disease include

• Maintaining a healthy weight

• Getting regular physical exercise

• Eating a balanced, low-fat diet

• Not smoking

• Controlling blood pressure and cholesterol

✔ **Know the warning signs for heart attack (see Chapter 5) and stroke (see Chapter 8).** Be prepared to go promptly to the hospital if you experience any of these signs.

✔ **Be proactive for your health.** *Proactive* may be an overworked buzzword these days, but it has two elements that I want to highlight for you:

• A can-do attitude

• A sense of taking control of events

One reason a diagnosis or potential diagnosis of heart disease is so frightening is that events seem out of your control. Regardless of what your heart health is at this moment, you can take control. Start by building your knowledge and being self-aware, healthwise (rather than ignoring possible warning signs).

You may want to start tuning in to your heart with the quiz in Chapter 1.

Going for a Checkup: The Medical History and Physical Examination

Regardless of whether you're going in for a regularly scheduled checkup, making an appointment with your primary-care physician, or being referred to a cardiologist to have a specific complaint examined, the doctor typically starts out with a number of important diagnostic techniques that may seem low-tech or simple to you. However, they provide an all-important road map for making a diagnosis, selecting further testing if needed, and planning treatment.

A seasoned primary-care physician or cardiologist knows that carefully observing and listening to the patient often provides more information than even the most advanced tests and that there's no substitute for an excellent history and comprehensive physical exam. Being ready to share your history and proactive about doing so can aid in your evaluation and diagnosis.

Taking your medical history

With any patient, I always begin by asking, "What brings you here?" The purpose in taking a patient's history is finding out as much as possible about the illness or symptoms that brought the individual to the doctor and about other factors in the patient's life that may affect his or her health. Here's the type of information a thorough history includes:

✔ History of the current illness, condition, and symptoms

✔ Current medications and dosages

✔ Past health history

✔ Family health history

✔ Social history, any factor that has bearing on physical and mental health, previous access to care, and so on, such as employment or economic status

Using hands before scans: The physical exam

Although you don't often think of the physical examination of the heart and vascular system as being a major test, it certainly is. For thousands of years, this venerable test has provided physicians with enormously important information to guide further evaluation of your heart.

"Sir, what ails you?"

How important is taking a patient's history to making a good diagnosis? A story that was part of the lore of Harvard Medical School when I was a student provides a telling answer:

Some years ago, a brilliant young woman med student — who was at the top of her class, a future Nobel laureate — was about to graduate with highest honors. Unheard of! Highest honors rarely were awarded, and with only the written and oral finals to complete, this woman was about to do it. The faculty hated the idea that it was even possible. If she didn't do well in her orals, the faculty thought, she wouldn't earn the summa cum laude designation.

As luck would have it, they had just the case on which to base the exam at the medical center — a patient with a very rare, esoteric condition that had baffled the best faculty minds and had taken batteries of tests to finally diagnose. The patient's condition was called paroxysmal nocturnal hematuria, PNH, which is sudden attacks in the night of blood in the urine. "We'll stump her," the faculty said. "We'll give her ten minutes with the patient and charts and ask her to diagnose the condition. She'll never do it, and we won't be able to award highest honors."

So they sent the young woman into the patient's room. In two minutes she was back in front of the surprised faculty. "Gentlemen," she said, "this patient can have only one thing, paroxysmal nocturnal hematuria." They were flabbergasted. "How did you do it? It took us weeks."

"Well," this gifted student said, "I went in and sat on the edge of his bed, took his hand in mine, and said, 'Sir, what ails you?' and he said, 'Paroxysmal nocturnal hematuria.'"

A good history is the only place to start. Be prepared to share yours.

"A good cardiologist must have the observational skills of Sherlock Holmes," someone once said, "the fine feeling in the hands of an expert safe-cracker, and the ears of a rabbit." Even if your cardiologist doesn't achieve these levels of expertise, the skills of *observation, palpation,* and *auscultation* remain the core of physical examination.

Observation

When you take your shirt off at the start of the cardiac physical examination, the astute physician begins with a series of observations and may look

- ✔ At the veins in your neck, which give an accurate estimate of the pressures of the venous system of the heart. A little fluttering actually occurs within the vein that provides further information concerning how the heart's booster pumps (the *atria*) are functioning.

- ✔ For any abnormal motions visible on the chest wall, which can suggest a variety of different cardiac conditions.

Palpation

After observation comes the laying on of hands — literally. The physician *palpates,* actually using fingertips to feel various cardiac structures. Two areas of interest are

- **Your neck:** The strength and characteristics of the pulses of the *carotid arteries,* the two large arteries on either side of the neck that supply the brain, provide plenty of useful information.

  - A normal carotid pulse suggests that the heart is pumping strongly and that no narrowing of either of these important conduits of brain food has occurred.

  - A weak *(parvus)* or delayed *(tardus)* pulse can suggest an obstruction to the outflow of blood from the heart, such as narrowing of the aortic valve or other obstructive condition.

  - An abnormal pulse (a *pulsus paradoxis*) can suggest that fluid has gathered in the sac around the heart or that severe lung disease may be present.

- **Your chest:** Palpating the front of the chest helps determine how well the main pumping chamber, the left ventricle, is pumping.

  - A normal left ventricle rises to meet the hand, rather like a firm handshake, and then rapidly falls away as it contracts.

  - Any differences in the feel of the left ventricle, such as a sustained grinding motion or a double impulse, can indicate either a thickened heart muscle or one that has been damaged.

Auscultation

Perhaps the most important part of the physical examination is *auscultation* — a fancy word that means the physician dons a stethoscope and listens to various heart sounds, such as these:

- **Lub-dub:** The sound of a normal heart. The first heart sound (affectionately known as *lub* and medically as *S1*) is caused by the closure of the valves between the ventricles and the atria to prevent blood from flowing backward into areas where it shouldn't go. The second heart sound *(dub or S2)* occurs at the end of the heart's contraction when valves between the ventricles and the arteries close to prevent blood from flowing back into the heart. During the intervals between these two sounds, the cardiologist listens for murmurs.

- **Swoosh:** Swoosh is not just the logo for a popular shoe manufacturer, it's also one sound made by abnormal blood flow.

Other abnormal heart sounds also have inventive descriptions. The typical murmur that occurs when the heart contracts (systole) is often characterized as the **chug** of an engine as it climbs a hill. The murmur that occurs when the heart is resting (diastole) often is described as the **whine** of the whistle of a train as it climbs a hill. (No, cardiologists are not graded on creativity.)

✔ **Extra heart sounds:** The cardiologist also listens for abnormal extra heart sounds known in cardiology as *gallops*. Gallops can occur as either a third heart sound (called S3) or a fourth heart sound (called S4). S3 comes after the lub-dub and has the timing of the *y* in *Kentucky*. Thus, the heart's rhythm goes S1=Ken, S2=tuck, S3=y. S4 comes before the lub-dub, with timing a bit like the *a* in the word *appendix*. Repeat these words quickly (that is, Kentucky, Kentucky, Kentucky), and you can tell why these sounds are called gallops. Cardiac abnormalities may also produce various *snaps* and *clicks*. For example, a mitral valve commonly produces a click when the valve prolapses (balloons backwards).

As simple as they seem (not a single digital display anywhere), these basic tools of observation, palpation, and auscultation of the heart often lead quickly toward an appropriate diagnosis and suggest which of an array of other cardiac tests need to be used to pinpoint a problem. I discuss these tests in Chapter 11.

The Checkup, Continued: Performing Clinical Laboratory Tests

"What do your lab tests indicate?" Veterans of regular checkups know that analyzing substances in blood or urine, for example, provides your doctors with a variety of useful signs and markers for many aspects of health.

The presence or absence of various substances in the blood can point to a number of different kinds of evidence about heart health and potential heart disease. Blood markers can be so useful, in fact, that identifying additional markers is an active medical research area. Blood test results also help physicians determine what additional testing procedures may be necessary. Finally, these kinds of tests are simple to do, cost-effective, and relatively easy on the patient. Here are some of the tests that your primary-care physician or cardiologist may use in evaluating your heart health.

Checking out common diagnostic blood tests

In a regular checkup or follow-up visit, your physician typically orders a variety of basic blood analyses that are performed using one or two vials of blood that are drawn after you've been fasting for 8 to 12 hours. Tests that directly relate to the heart and cardiovascular system include the following:

- **Lipid profile or lipid panel:** This test is an analysis of cholesterol, HDL and LDL cholesterol, and triglycerides (see Chapter 14).

- **Complete blood count (CBC):** This test provides an analysis of various components of the blood, such as red and white blood cells. The CBC is used to diagnose anemia and to point to the need for other tests.

- **Glucose level:** This test serves as an analysis of insulin resistance. Because insulin resistance and diabetes are risk factors for CAD, your physician closely monitors this result.

- **A basic or comprehensive metabolic panel:** This test provides an analysis of various factors related to kidney function, liver function, and electrolytes, which can be related to heart disease.

- **Thyroid level:** Your physician monitors this test for evidence of an overactive thyroid, because such a condition can cause your heart to beat too rapidly.

Stepping up to specialized diagnostic blood tests

If you're at higher risk of heart disease, already have a heart problem, or earlier lab test results indicate a need for further testing, your physician may order specialized tests such as the following:

- **High sensitivity C-reactive protein (hs-CRP):** This analysis detects inflammation in the blood vessels. Other inflammatory markers that your physician may choose to check include levels of *fibrinogen* or *ferritin,* two other blood proteins.

- **Homocysteine:** A high level of homocysteine is linked to increased risk of heart disease. This test provides another measure that your physician may want to use in addition to a lipid profile.

✔ **Prothrombin time:** This test analyzes the amount of time required for your blood to clot and helps physicians regulate drugs used to keep platelets from clumping (aspirin is one) and to keep blood from clotting (warfarin — Coumadin — is a common one).

✔ **BNP level:** If you have severe shortness of breath, one of the symptoms of heart failure (see Chapter 7), your physician may want to check the level of *B-type natriuretic peptide* (BNP), a protein that is secreted to ease strain on the heart.

✔ **Cardiac enzymes:** Elevated levels of these proteins can indicate whether your heart muscle has suffered damage, as in a heart attack.

Screening with Other Tests

During a regular checkup, your physician may want to take an electrocardiogram (ECG or EKG), which records the heart's electrical impulses, and perhaps even administer an exercise tolerance test.

Using all these basic evaluations — history, physical, lab tests, and ECG — your doctor monitors your heart health and the progress of any manifestation of heart disease. Based on these observations and results, your doctor may recommend further diagnostic testing using a variety of more high-tech procedures that I discuss in detail in Chapter 11.

Chapter 11

Using Diagnostic Tests

*I*n the war against heart disease, cardiologists have a number of amazing tools, simple and high-tech, at their disposal. Thousands of times a day, patients undergo various forms of cardiac testing in every major medical setting and cardiologist's office in the United States. The results of these tests yield significant information that helps doctors work with people to maintain healthy hearts or diagnose ailing hearts.

Cardiac testing, however, can also be frightening and intimidating for patients. Physicians often speak a lingo all their own and forget to explain adequately to the patient the reason for each test. In addition, strange machinery and equipment can jangle already tense nerves.

This chapter briefly explains most common cardiac tests and demystifies the reasons for each of them. Although I refer to these tests in various chapters throughout this book, you can use this chapter as an overview for ready reference.

Diagnosing Heart Disease with Noninvasive Tests

From the more-than-a-century-old electrocardiogram, to echocardiography, to the latest high-tech magnetic resonance imaging (MRI), noninvasive diagnostic tests provide information about what's going right and what's going wrong with your heart.

Electrocardiogram

Invented more than 100 years ago, the *electrocardiogram* (also called ECG or EKG) represents cardiology's first high-tech tool. But this graphic recording of the heart's electrical impulses remains one of the most useful tests. Many doctors include it as part of a routine annual physical exam to assess any potential heart problems. Moreover, the ECG is an early diagnostic step taken when an individual exhibits symptoms that may represent heart disease.

How it works

Measuring the heart's electrical impulses requires the placement of a number of electrical sensors (leads) in specific and strategic positions on the chest, arms, and legs. Because this test is administered while the heart is at rest, you're asked to lie down while electrical information from the sensors is gathered simultaneously. Data from the sensors is recorded as a graph. The entire process is very easy and comfortable.

What it shows

Astute clinicians know that the graphic tracings of the heart's electrical activity can reveal

- Evidence of a heart attack
- Occurrence of angina or unstable angina during the test
- Information about the entire electrical conduction system and rhythm of the heart
- Evidence of thickening in the heart wall
- Evidence of enlarged chambers, such as the atria
- Problems in the pericardium (the sac around the heart)

Exercise tolerance test

The *exercise tolerance test* (ETT — also called an *exercise stress test*) is an electrocardiogram that's administered while the heart is beating fast during exercise. After you're properly wired up, you're asked to walk and/or run at progressively higher speeds on a motorized treadmill or pedal against steadily increasing resistance on a stationary cycle. These exercise activities cause the heart to speed up.

The two basic types of exercise tolerance tests are

✔ A *maximal* exercise tolerance test, during which the patient is asked to exercise to the maximum degree possible

✔ A *submaximal* exercise tolerance test, during which the test is stopped before the individual achieves maximal exercise

Among the most important clinical information that this test reveals is whether adequate blood flow is reaching the heart during exercise. Thus, the exercise tolerance test is extremely useful in making the diagnosis of coronary artery disease (CAD), angina, and in some instances, unstable angina. As an added bonus, your doctor can estimate your cardiovascular fitness (also called your *aerobic capacity*) based on the amount of exercise that you're able to do on the exercise tolerance test.

Holter monitoring

When a patient complains of significant *palpitation* (see Chapter 6), the cardiologist often orders a 24-hour monitor that records every heartbeat during an entire 24-hour period to determine whether serious rhythm problems are occurring. This form of electrocardiogram is called *Holter monitoring.* You're asked to wear a small device attached to a belt around your waist and attached to electrical leads on your chest.

Cardiac event monitoring

When a patient's rhythm problems don't occur frequently enough to be recorded by a Holter monitor, the cardiologist may order a cardiac event monitor. This monitor is a small device that you wear and activate when the arrhythmia occurs. You may either hold the device to your chest during the event or the device may have leads that stay attached to your chest — similar to the Holter monitor. Implantable cardiac event recorders that can record events up to 24 months also are available.

Echocardiography

For cardiac medicine, as for the navy, an echo is often just the thing! In much the same way that an echo helps navy ships find out (by using sonar) what's lurking beneath them, an echo helps cardiologists find what's lurking inside the ribcages of their patients by using an echocardiogram. In fact, with the exception of the ECG, echocardiography is perhaps the most widely used noninvasive procedure in cardiovascular medicine.

How it works

An *echocardiogram,* which also goes by the names *cardiac sonogram* and *cardiac ultrasound,* bounces sound waves off various structures of the heart. Sound waves are sent out by and then return to a device known as a transducer. The transducer measures the reflected sound waves, converting them into a moving picture of all the structures of the heart.

In some cases, a cardiologist may order a *transesophageal echocardiogram* (TEE), a test in which the transducer is passed through the mouth and into the esophagus near the heart — a position that produces extremely clear pictures of the heart's structures.

What it shows

Among its many uses, echocardiography is used for evaluating

- Whether any of the heart's four valves are narrowed *(stenosed)* or leaking *(regurgitation)* and how well replacement and reconstructed valves are working after surgery

- How well the heart is pumping

- Blockage of blood flow *(ischemia)* in the coronary arteries related to CAD when used in a drug-simulated stress test (dobutamine stress echocardiography)

- Whether any major damage has occurred either to the heart muscles or the structures around the heart

- The existence of congenital heart disease

High-resolution carotid ultrasound can provide useful information about the walls of the carotid arteries in your neck. Certain characteristics of the walls of these major vessels have been strongly associated with CAD. Thus, carotid ultrasound has gained an increasing following as a noninvasive way of estimating the risk of developing CAD.

Magnetic resonance imaging (MRI)

You may be more familiar with *magnetic resonance imaging* (MRI) as it relates to sports medicine and diagnosing injuries to joints, muscles, and connective tissue (such as cartilage); however, with advances in technology, MRIs have gained widespread use in cardiology.

How it works

MRI uses large magnets to create a powerful magnetic field that can form computerized images of the heart without using X-rays. Most MRI equipment uses a moving platform positioned within a circular or enclosed tunnel that looks a bit like a large doughnut. The tunnel is part of a larger mechanism that houses the magnets that create (noisily, I might add) the magnetic field. Newer, open MRI equipment has been developed, however — an innovation welcomed by the claustrophobic.

What it shows

Magnetic resonance imaging produces three-dimension pictures of the heart that show

- The heart muscle and the pericardium (sac surrounding it)
- Areas damaged by a heart attack
- The condition of the aorta, helping to identify dissection or aneurysm in that structure
- Certain congenital defects

Evidence from recent research suggests the MRI may also be extremely useful in determining the composition of fatty plaques in coronary arteries, which may lead to early, precise diagnosis of CAD.

Computed tomography (CT)

Actually, computers are used in almost every type of diagnostic test today. But one particular type of scan, *computed tomography,* typically is referred to as computerized imaging. If I said "CT scan" or "CAT scan," you'd know immediately what I mean, right? You can't put a medical drama or documentary on TV without the requisite CT scan. With continual advances in precision and versatility, such as very high-speed CT, tomography has developed into increasingly important applications for diagnosing and monitoring heart disease.

CT scanning combines the power of X-ray images with computer processing to present images of a variety of cardiac structures in a cross-sectional format.

How it works

The patient lies on a platform that can be positioned inside a large, circular X-ray machine that looks a bit like a huge doughnut. The shape of the machinery enables it to produce images from all sides. The platform moves the patient slowly past the X-ray beam, which rotates 360 degrees and enables the computer to record multiple cross-sectional *slices,* or *slides,* of the patient's body.

What it shows

The CT scan creates images of the heart, large vessels leading to the heart, and other structures in the chest, such as the lungs.

With the advent of new, high-speed, multislice CT scanners, determining the amount of calcium that's accumulated in the coronary arteries is now possible. The calcium is an indication of *chronic atherosclerosis* (clogging of the arteries). Finding calcium in the coronary arteries is useful in the early, precise diagnosis of CAD.

Electron-beam computed tomography (EBCT scan) is another newer type of very fast CT that uses a tiny electron-beam X-ray to produce precise images of the structures of the heart. It also is useful in measuring the amount of calcium in the coronary arteries.

Which type of advanced CT scan your cardiologist orders usually is a function of the kind of equipment that's available in the medical or diagnostic center where you go to have the tests.

Invasive versus noninvasive testing

If you hear your cardiologist mutter something about an invasive procedure, don't panic. You won't need the nearest emergency bunker. Tests and procedures in cardiac medicine are broadly classified as *noninvasive* and *invasive.* As the names suggest, noninvasive tests, such as electrocardiograms, echocardiograms, and computed tomography (CT) scans, are the kind in which the body literally is not invaded. Invasive procedures, on the other hand, involve actually putting instruments inside the body or invading it. Invasive procedures include cardiac catheterization, angioplasty, and electrophysiology exams. Thanks to modern anesthesia, invasive procedures can be administered with little or no discomfort.

Diagnosing Heart Disease Using Nuclear Imaging

Invasive cardiologists (who spend most of their time doing heart catheterization and angioplasty) used to joke that *nuclear* medicine was really *unclear* medicine. In fact, various nuclear techniques provide extremely valuable information about how the heart's functioning and whether blood flow is adequate. Several techniques combine computed tomography with nuclear imaging. The term *nuclear* indicates that the tests make use of a radioactive tracer material that's injected into the bloodstream to create a more precise image of the flow of blood through the heart and cardiovascular system.

Single photon emission computed tomography (SPECT)

A s*ingle photon emission computed tomography* (SPECT) scan of the heart provides very clear three-dimensional pictures of a functioning heart.

How it works

During a SPECT scan, a radionuclide tracer (a radioactive substance) is injected into the bloodstream. As it flows through the structures that are being scanned, including the heart, the tracer releases energy that's recorded by a camera sensitive to the gamma rays emitted by the radionuclide tracer. Those images are then compiled by a computer.

What it shows

SPECT scans provide a relatively cost-effective and minimally invasive way of measuring how blood is flowing through the heart by looking at areas of the heart muscle that are not receiving adequate blood flow during stress and rest phases. The results of a SPECT scan may also indicate the need for additional testing.

SPECT scans also help doctors make a better diagnosis of heart disease in women, for whom ECGs and ETTs are not nearly as accurate as they are for men. They're also useful in evaluating heart disease in certain diabetic patients who cannot tolerate an exercise stress test.

Two types of SPECT tests merit specific mention:

- **Gated blood pool scanning:** In this test, which is also called *RVG* or *MUGA* scanning, a radioactive tracer is placed in the bloodstream and circulates through the heart while pictures of the heart are taken. This test enables cardiologists to estimate how well the heart is pumping.

- **Nuclear stress test:** In this test, *thallium* or *technetium* is injected into a vein. This radioactive tracer travels to the coronary arteries and ultimately is carried by the blood to the heart tissue. The test provides pictures of the heart before, during, and after physical stress. The degree to which the tracer reaches various parts of the heart provides a good estimate of how blood is flowing through the coronary arteries.

Positron emission tomography (PET)

Positron emission tomography (PET) scans can provide precise information about blood flow to cardiac structures. Because the technique and the equipment used to perform PET testing are quite expensive and sophisticated, it is available in only a limited number of centers in the U.S.

How it works

A PET scan, in many cases, uses a two-step process. First, an initial scan takes place with the patient resting on a table that slips through the scanning device. Then, radioactive material (a tracer) is injected into the patient. As the tracer enters the bloodstream and reaches the heart it releases energy as gamma rays. Machines known as *photomultiplier-scintillator detectors* record these rays. A computer then analyzes the recordings to produce a three-dimensional image. Sometimes a second scan is performed while the patient is exercising. An advantage of the PET scan is that results are more reliable because certain body structures or conditions such as obesity or large breasts do not distort the images, which often happens with other types of scanning.

What it shows

PET scans are useful in diagnosing CAD and assessing the functioning of the heart muscle. For example, a PET scan may be used after a heart attack to identify areas of the heart muscle that are damaged but still able to recover. It also can provide information about oxygen consumption and glucose metabolism by the heart and about concentrations of other substances.

Plumbing 101: Diagnosing Heart Disease Using Heart Catheterization

Cardiac or *heart catheterization* (cath) is an invasive procedure in which the cardiologist inserts a small plastic tube, or *catheter,* into a large vein or artery in the leg or arm and guides it into the heart or coronary arteries. Heart catheterization can be used to perform various diagnostic tests and treatment procedures.

It may give you a chuckle to know that within the profession these invasive cardiologists (I'm one of them) are called *plumbers* because they work on the pipes (the coronary arteries) and the pump (the heart).

Angiography

When a contrast material (often called a *dye*) is injected through the catheter to make arteries or other structures of the heart visible to X-rays, the procedure is called *angiography.* An advanced procedure, it usually is performed in a heart catheterization laboratory by a cardiologist who specializes in the field. Patients undergo heart catheterizations to determine pressures in the heart and to provide definitive evidence of any abnormalities that may be present either in the pumping chamber itself or the arteries that supply it with blood. As a practical matter, cardiologists can catheterize either the left side of the heart or the side of the right heart individually or, as often occurs, perform both procedures sequentially while the patient is in the heart catheterization lab.

Left heart catheterization

The cardiologist typically inserts the catheter into arterial circulation through the *femoral artery* in the groin, and then threads it up into either the left heart pumping chamber or individually into each of the three arteries that supply the heart. Contrast material then is injected and pictures (angiograms) of the blood flow are taken. Patients usually undergo a left heart catheterization to determine pressures and to take pictures of the left heart and the coronary arteries that supply it to determine the amount of blockage or CAD present. Virtually all patients who undergo *coronary artery bypass grafting* and all patients who undergo *angioplasty* undergo heart catheterization first. (For more information regarding these procedures, see Chapter 16.)

Right heart catheterization

The cardiologist inserts the catheter into the venous circulation in the *femoral vein in the leg* and threads it up into the right atrium and from there into the right ventricle and then out into the pulmonary artery, recording pressures — as shown in Figure 11-1 — along the way. This procedure typically reveals how the right heart, which pumps blood to the lungs, is functioning. Occasionally it is done to determine whether any congenital abnormalities exist, such as a hole in the muscular walls (the septa) that separate the right and left atria and right and left ventricles. Such holes, which are known as *atrial septal defects* (ASD) or *ventricular septal defects* (VSD), are relatively rare conditions that usually must be repaired surgically.

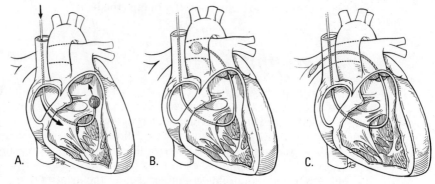

Figure 11-1:
Right heart catheter-ization.

A.   B.   C.

Checking out electrical problems in the heart

On the basis of the results of an electrocardiogram (ECG) or other evaluation, some heart rhythm problems may require the most advanced test of the heart's electric company, an *electrophysiology study,* or *EP study.*

How it works

An EP study takes place in a specialized laboratory that's similar to a heart catheterization lab. Specialized catheters are inserted through a vein or artery and appropriately positioned within the heart to measure targeted electrical activity and pathways. The catheter also can be used to trigger certain arrhythmias within a controlled setting to evaluate problems or treatments. In some cases, it may be used to administer treatment, called *catheter ablation* (see Chapter 16), right after the evaluation is made. EP studies typically are performed in large hospital centers by specially trained cardiologists whose field is *electrophysiology.*

What it shows

EP studies are used to

- ✔ Diagnose arrhythmias such as bradycardias or tachycardias
- ✔ Provide more accurate diagnoses of some sinus node problems (see Chapter 6)
- ✔ Confirm the presence of AV block (see Chapter 6)
- ✔ Help determine heart-related causes of fainting
- ✔ Determine whether a pacemaker or implanted defibrillator is needed

Monitoring heart performance and pressure in the hospital

The heart function of almost every patient in a coronary care unit (CCU) receives constant monitoring, whether it's for diagnosing a heart problem or checking the results of heart surgery. Several procedures that monitor heart performance and pressure in these circumstances make use of catheterization.

- ✔ **Arterial catheterization:** A small tube (catheter) is placed into a branch of the arterial system to monitor the blood pressure and the level of oxygenation in the arterial circulation accurately. Although such *arterial catheters* (also called *arterial lines* or *A lines*) may be put into any artery, the most common is the artery on the thumb side of the wrist.

- ✔ **Central venous catheterization:** When delivering potent medications, having access to the deep venous system is often necessary. A long catheter is threaded through the neck, groin, or arm into this part of the venous system and up near the right side of the heart so that medications can be delivered efficiently and pressures within the venous system can be measured accurately. This procedure frequently is used in the CCU for measuring the *central venous pressure* (CVP).

- ✔ **Pulmonary artery catheterization:** The pulmonary artery is the main vessel leading out into the lungs from the right ventricle. It carries deoxygenated blood to the lungs where it is reoxygenated. The pressures in pulmonary arterial circulation often are extremely useful in determining therapies for the patient. Thus, this procedure uses a thin catheter that is inserted into a vein and threaded into the right atrium, through the right ventricle, and out into the pulmonary artery, enabling cardiologists to accurately measure pressure in the right and left sides of the heart. (Check out Figure 11-1.)

Chapter 12

Forming a Partnership with Your Doctor

*I*n the words of comedienne Joan Rivers, "Can we talk?" Talking, of course, is exactly what you and your doctor need to do. Throughout this book, one of my mantras has been "forming a partnership with your physician." Fighting so serious a foe as heart disease is not a battle to take on by yourself. But finding the right physician in the mazes of the medical system is not always easy and neither is knowing how to establish clear lines of communication and cooperation. Hence, I've written this chapter. Think of it as a primer on partnership.

Building a Solid Health-Care Partnership

Like all partnerships — whether business relationships, marriages, or friendships — patient-physician partnerships must be based on open communication and trust. At its best, a partnership between you and your physician can be a long-term, trusting relationship with benefits to your cardiovascular health. Discussing how to optimize your cardiovascular health with your physician also should be a pleasure to which you and your doctor look forward. Many doctors, it pains me to say, are not willing, able, or ready to accept this kind of a partnership with their patients. But I believe that every patient needs to be a good consumer. That means you need to have realistic goals and realistically high expectations when selecting and working with a personal physician and, if you need one, a cardiologist.

Of course, your health-care choices extend beyond finding the right primary-care physician, so I offer tips for choosing a managed-care plan and a hospital, as well.

Selecting a primary-care doctor

Almost invariably, people, even those who have heart disease, depend upon their primary-care doctor for most of their health-care needs. I've always been surprised by how randomly many people choose a physician. You need to regard your physician as a consultant in the same way you regard your accountant or your lawyer, and take the same care in choosing him or her.

First, look for a doctor who has superior knowledge about medicine, who listens, who asks pertinent questions, and who provides useful explanations and answers. Also look for a physician who displays genuine concern, cost-consciousness, and a determination to keep working on *any* medical problem that you have. Above all, your doctor needs to be someone who cares about you and inspires confidence, optimism, and hope in you.

A good way to begin identifying such candidates is by asking neighbors, family, or friends for recommendations. You can also obtain information or referrals by contacting local hospitals, medical schools, or medical societies. Many hospitals, clinics, and private practices now have Web sites where you likewise can obtain basic information.

Narrow down your choice to two or three physician candidates and then call their offices to arrange a time to speak with them, either in person or on the phone. This important preinterview enables you to find out how the physician approaches the world and his or her patients. Here are some questions you may want to ask during the preinterview:

- ✔ Where did you go to medical school?
- ✔ Where did you train after medical school?
- ✔ What are your special areas of medical interest?
- ✔ Can you tell me a little bit about how you approach medicine and patient care?

If you have an existing cardiac condition, ask the candidates about their backgrounds in and knowledge of your particular condition and what they think about lifestyle factors such as exercise and nutrition. Asking what they think about mind/body connections and supplements may also be worthwhile. (Be careful when asking these questions, because some of the very best physicians may be thrown off-guard by them, at least until they get to know you better.)

Asking about practical matters also is a good idea. Questions such as "Which insurance plans does your practice accept?" and "At which hospitals do you have admitting privileges?" reveal a great deal about your physician candidate. The answer to the latter question is particularly important because the best physicians almost inevitably have admitting privileges at the best hospitals.

When you're considering the answers to your questions and just how the conversation went in general, don't forget that who you are as an individual plays a role of utmost importance in deciding which doctor is best for you. Some people like detailed and thorough explanations. Others want a more regimented approach with less specific information. Don't be embarrassed to interview a few physicians to find out whether they fit best with who you are. Remember, you're establishing a long-term partnership here, so you should not rush into it.

Finding the right cardiologist

If you already have heart disease, you're going to be best cared for by both your family doctor and a cardiologist. A cardiologist has advanced training in *cardiology,* which is a subspecialty of internal medicine. Pursuing such a subspecialty typically means anywhere from three to five years of training in addition to full training in internal medicine.

Choosing a cardiologist can be a little trickier than choosing a family care doctor, because the normal sources of information — family and friends — may not be as familiar with cardiology specialists, or you may belong to an insurance or managed-care plan that requires you to select from a particular group of physicians or to be referred by your primary-care physician. You can, however, begin your search by asking your primary-care physician these questions about the cardiologists he or she recommends:

✔ Where did the cardiologist train?

✔ What are his or her areas of specialty within cardiology?

✔ At what hospitals does the cardiologist practice?

✔ How does the cardiologist approach his or her patients?

✔ Is the cardiologist willing to form partnerships and talk to patients, rather than merely giving directions and demanding that they be followed?

✔ How accessible is the cardiologist?

✔ How is the cardiologist as a human being?

On the basis of this information, you may then want to interview two or three cardiologists in much the same way that you interviewed your primary-care doctor.

Choosing and working with a managed-care plan

In this day and age, almost half of Americans get their basic medical care through some form of managed-care plan, whether it's an HMO (health-maintenance organization), PPO (preferred-provider organization), or some other member of the Alphabet City of managed care.

If you receive your insurance through your employer, the way many Americans do, you may even be offered a choice of plans or choices within a single plan. If so, don't make the common mistake of basing your choice solely on cost. (That isn't how you chose your car, is it?) Instead, look carefully at these issues:

✔ Access to the physicians you want to see

✔ The qualifications of the physicians who have chosen the plan

✔ The hospitals that are affiliated with the plan

✔ Logistical issues such as convenience of doctors and hospitals to you

✔ If you have an established cardiac condition, the availability of certain treatments through the managed-care plan

Your human resources professional at work should be able to help you sort through these issues. Most managed-care plans have their own Web sites, so you can search the Internet for information on each plan.

If you must provide your own health insurance, you may have a more difficult time finding an affordable plan that gives you the coverage you want. Check with friends who are self-employed and with insurance agents when you have to choose an individual plan. A group or organization to which you belong may also offer its members some form of group insurance. Do an online search for possibilities. Again, be sure to get the answers you need. Having an existing condition, such as cardiovascular disease, affects what coverage you can obtain.

Hunting down a hospital

Choosing a hospital is a surprisingly important health-care decision, particularly when you have cardiac disease. Recent studies show that patients at certain hospitals tend to have better outcomes. As a general rule, these hospitals are the ones that have programs for physicians in training. If your primary-care physician or cardiologist plans to refer you to a hospital for advanced testing or surgery, don't be shy about asking about the hospital's expertise and experience with these procedures. If I were facing open-heart surgery, for instance, I'd surely want to be in the care of a hospital team that specializes in that kind of surgery, performs it frequently (like every day!), and has an outstanding record of success and care.

If you already have established heart disease, I advise you to choose a large hospital with experience in cardiac care and a training program, if possible. Within medicine, these hospitals typically are *tertiary care hospitals,* which means they specialize in caring for patients with many advanced illnesses, including severe forms of heart disease. These hospitals usually can be identified through local medical societies or local or regional medical schools in your area.

Establishing a Partnership with Your Physician

Establishing an effective partnership between you and your physician requires four key elements.

✔ **Communication:** Open communication, the foundation of partnership, is clearly a two-way street.

- You have the right to expect your physician to fully and openly give you the information that helps you understand your condition and participate in your treatment.

- By the same token, your physician has the right to expect you to be frank about the symptoms you're experiencing, not only from your condition but also from any medicines you're taking.

✔ **Trust:** Trust enables both communication and commitment in partnership. You must trust that your physician always has your best interests at heart and that your physician is competent, caring, and concerned about your well-being. By the same token, your physician has to be able to trust that you're committed to your own well-being.

✔ **Commitment to the treatment plan:** Your responsibility within the partnership is to be committed to a treatment plan that you and your doctor agree upon. You shouldn't agree to a treatment plan unless you intend to carry it out.

You also need to be committed to finding out all that you can about your condition and the whys and wherefores of various treatment procedures. Ask again if you don't understand something. Ask your doctor for information. Use reputable print and online resources (such as the ones recommended throughout this book) to educate yourself. The more informed and knowledgeable you are, the more committed and equal a partner you're likely to be.

✔ **Quality care:** Your physician bears responsibility for quality care, not only as a function of his or her knowledge and integrity but also as a function of the total medical-care system serving you. Ensuring that any other physicians involved in your care also practice quality care is your physician's responsibility. All of the facilities associated with that system — including the office and the hospital and the performance of all the individuals within those settings — ultimately are the responsibility of the physician.

Communication and trust are elements shared between you and your doctor. Commitment to a treatment plan is your domain, and the quality of your care is your physician's.

Identifying what you have a right to expect of your physician

As a consumer, you have the right to expect that your physician will

✔ Listen carefully and provide thorough, clear explanations for procedures, conditions, and treatment options

✔ Answer your questions

✔ Possess the skills and knowledge of a physician committed to ongoing medical education and at the cutting edge of medical science

If your physician is not meeting these expectations, then it's time to look for another doctor.

Looking at what your physician has a right to expect of you

Yes, we docs have the right to some expectations, too. I can tell you, as a physician, nothing is more frustrating than trying to control blood pressure in someone who intermittently takes their medicine or trying to control blood lipids for patients who don't pay attention to even the basics of sound nutrition and decreasing the amount of fat they eat. You need to be your own best friend when it comes to your own medical care.

Your commitment is so important that I'm going to reemphasize these points:

- ✔ If you have reservations or doubts about the treatment plan your doctor proposes, discuss these problems fully with your physician before agreeing to the plan.

- ✔ After you agree upon a plan, do it — and stick to it. If any problems, symptoms, or side effects arise, tell your doctor. Pick up the phone and tell the receptionist or nurse (whoever serves as the gatekeeper for incoming calls) exactly why you need to talk to the doctor.

- ✔ Be sure to follow the lifestyle measures. Treatment is more than just taking a prescribed medication.

- ✔ Don't ever be ashamed to share your problems with your doctor. Nothing is shameful about having difficulties with making changes in your life. It is hard, but it is possible. You need the kind of relationship with your doctor that enables you to talk about your problems and not feel ashamed.

- ✔ Educate yourself about your condition.

Helping your primary-care doctor and cardiologist communicate

Although this topic may seem like a strange one to include, communication between your primary-care doctor and cardiologist is important. You're probably already thinking, "Shouldn't my doctors work with each other as a matter of course?" Naturally, they try their best to do that, but I can tell you that many times lab values and other critical information are lost, even in the best systems between the best doctors.

Tips for asking the right questions

Here are some recommended questions that you can ask your doctor about any condition that he or she may discover during an evaluation. You may even want to copy this list to take with you.

✔ What is my diagnosis?

✔ What tests will I need to undergo?

✔ Are there any side effects or dangers to these tests?

✔ What is the recommended treatment?

✔ What are the potential side effects of the treatment?

✔ Are there any treatment choices?

✔ Are there any other questions that I should be asking?

✔ Is there any source of information that I can read about my diagnosis?

You can play an important role as a fail-safe communication link between your primary-care physician and your cardiologist. One way to accomplish this goal is making sure that the notes that go into your physician's record also are sent to you. Such notes include not only the impression of your progress from your primary-care doctor and your cardiologist but also any pertinent findings and laboratory values. Your medical record, by the way, is a legal document that belongs to you.

Optimizing office visits

Office visits to the doctor are a pain, aren't they? Particularly when you have to go out of town. So here are some tips for getting the most out of them.

✔ **Be efficient.** Respect your physician's time and expect that your physician will respect your time, too. If forms need to be completed, try to arrive a little early. Bring notes that track your symptoms and, if you've been referred by a primary-care physician, try to bring copies of pertinent medical records and lab tests. Bring a written list of the medications that you're taking, including the frequency and dosage. If you have a discharge summary from a hospitalization, share it with your physician, particularly a subspecialist such as a cardiologist. If you need to cancel your appointment, common courtesy mandates that you try to do so as early as possible. (The same goes for the physician.)

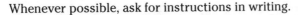

✔ **Describe your symptoms.** Be prepared to tell your doctor about any symptoms that you have, when they occur, how severe they are, and how they affect you.

✔ **Bring notes.** Seeing your notes about the issues that you have always is beneficial to a physician, so write down your questions ahead of time. (That doesn't mean you can't also ask new ones as they arise.)

✔ **Ask about your diagnosis.** Asking specifically about your likely diagnosis and what tests the physician regards as important for specifically pinning down that diagnosis is important. Don't be afraid to ask for this information in layman's terms.

✔ **Take notes.** Many times, patients leave the doctor's office and forget what they discussed. Visiting the doctor often is stressful, so don't be afraid to take notes during the discussion and, for that matter, bring someone with you. A second pair of ears helps. Absent that, you can also use a tape recorder.

Whenever possible, ask for instructions in writing.

✔ **Schedule a follow-up appointment.** If a follow-up appointment is necessary, ask the doctor specifically when to schedule it. Asking how to reach the physician in case of an emergency also is important.

Making testing easier

Most of us at some time face testing either to confirm a diagnosis or assess the efficacy of treatment. Wandering through a maze of unfamiliar hospital halls, chart and referral slip in hand, can be frightening and confusing. Avoid such anxiety and confusion by planning ahead.

✔ Ask your primary-care physician or your cardiologist exactly what tests you'll be undergoing and what the potential benefit and outcome of each of the tests or procedures will be.

✔ Ask for a map and/or directions to the testing center or hospital. If your physician's office doesn't have this information, call the testing center for directions and be sure to find out where to park and where to check in.

✔ Ask the technicians at each testing or procedure area exactly what will happen during the test, any side effects that you may feel, and what information the test is likely to reveal. Most technicians and physicians are delighted to explain their procedures.

Considering Special Issues in the Doctor-Patient Relationship

I've outlined some general rules for working with your physician. However, a few special circumstances may come up that you need to consider. The following sections look at a few of them.

Participating in research studies

Many physicians today are involved in clinical research. Most participate in these studies to further their knowledge and to keep up with modern medical advances. For the most part, clinical research is a good thing. Unfortunately, a few unscrupulous physicians engage in clinical research for monetary gain and sometimes pressure patients to enter research projects that may not be of benefit to them.

If your physician recommends that you enter a clinical research trial, you have the right to ask whether the therapy being studied has any recognized benefits. You also have the right to have a thorough explanation of why this therapy is being recommended and how it differs from regular therapy. Although I support clinical research, I think it is important that patients not be coerced (even subtly) into participating in clinical research trials — particularly when up-to-date therapies are established in almost every aspect of cardiovascular disease.

Getting your physician's attention when it's difficult

Nothing is more frustrating than having your physician ignore you when you have questions, concerns, or troubling symptoms. Unfortunately, many physician's offices screen calls in such a way that it's difficult to get through to the physician. Often an assistant, such as a nurse, takes your question, confers with the doctor, and calls you back. If you feel your concerns have been handled appropriately by this "physician extender," that's okay. If not, specifically request that the physician call you back to address your concern. If the physician is unwilling to do so after several phone calls, then write the physician a letter saying that you're concerned about his or her failure to call you back in a timely manner. If the doctor also ignores the written request, then it's time to look for a new physician. After all, would you accept that kind of treatment from your lawyer or accountant?

Getting a second opinion

You have a right to obtain a second opinion about any serious diagnosis. Second opinions are deeply respected in medicine. A good physician will never be offended if you seek a second opinion. After all, in many instances, two heads are better than one. Don't be embarrassed to ask your physician to recommend someone to offer a second opinion. If your physician is the kind of doctor that you want to see, he or she will have no problem with this straightforward request.

Changing to a new doctor when necessary

Switching physicians also is completely within your rights as a patient. Different patient and physician styles often do not mesh perfectly, which can hinder your ability to communicate adequately. You also need to trust that your physician has superior medical skills and knowledge. If you don't feel confident in either of these areas, it's time to start looking for another physician.

One word of caution: As you're considering the need to change, examine your own thinking and emotions for signs of denial. Sometimes when a physician gives a diagnosis that is difficult to accept, a patient may have the inclination to start looking around for a doctor who will offer a more comfortable, if less truthful, diagnosis. All too often, such "doctor shopping" leads to inferior care.

Part IV
Controlling and Treating Heart Disease

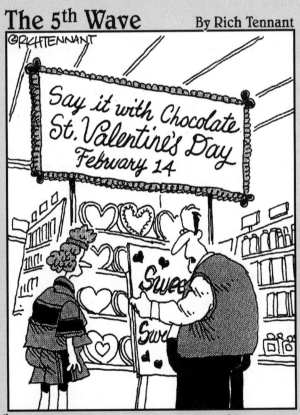

The 5th Wave   By Rich Tennant

Say it with Chocolate
St. Valentine's Day
February 14

"Of course you're better off eating grains and vegetables, but for St. Valentine's Day, we've never been very successful with 'Say it with Legumes'."

In this part . . .

Get a grip on what you need to know to control two conditions that are major contributing causes of heart disease: high blood pressure and elevated cholesterol. Then, take a look at the most common drug and medical treatments (short of invasive or surgical procedures) that are available to physicians for treating various heart problems. Finally, check out some of the most common invasive procedures, such as angioplasty, and surgical procedures, such as coronary bypass grafting, that are used to treat heart problems.

Chapter 13

Combating High Blood Pressure

- -

In This Chapter

▶ Understanding high blood pressure and its relationship to other diseases

▶ Linking high blood pressure to lifestyle and genetic issues

▶ Lowering blood pressure with lifestyle modifications

▶ Partnering with your physician to combat high blood pressure

- -

*H*igh blood pressure, or *hypertension,* is quite common in the United States. More than one-fourth of the adult population — more than 50 million people — suffer from high blood pressure. Furthermore, as you grow older, you're more likely to have high blood pressure. At some point, almost everyone will develop high blood pressure. But don't despair. In partnership with your physician, you fortunately can take great strides to prevent high blood pressure in the first place and to control it if you get it. And, in so doing, you can lower your risk of heart disease, kidney failure, stroke, and many other serious conditions associated with poorly controlled hypertension. An added bonus: You'll benefit from enhanced physical well-being, and you'll probably enjoy life more, too.

Understanding Hypertension: The Silent Killer

Hypertension is called *The Silent Killer,* because it typically does not cause any noticeable symptoms. The result:

✔ Almost 29 percent of adults in the United States have high blood pressure.

✔ Many people aren't even aware that they have high blood pressure. In fact, more than 30 percent of people with hypertension don't know it.

✔ Many more know they have high blood pressure but aren't being treated.

✔ Others are being treated but still don't have their blood pressure under good control. Among persons taking medication, only 53 percent have their blood pressure effectively controlled. Among all persons with high blood pressure, 69 percent do not have it controlled.

✔ More than 50 percent of the people with high blood pressure aren't being treated at all.

But it doesn't have to be that way. The medical profession and people with high blood pressure have enormous room for improvement in combating hypertension. The place to start is with a little education.

Defining blood pressure

As the heart pumps blood through the circulatory system, the blood that's being pumped exerts pressure against the interior walls of the blood vessels. Your *blood pressure* reading consists of two measurements of the pressure exerted on the walls of the arteries. These measurements are expressed in millimeters (mm) of mercury (Hg). For example, 110mm/70 mm Hg (read "one-ten over seventy millimeters of mercury") or 120/80 mm Hg are two typical readings for *normal blood pressure.* The top or higher number is called the *systolic pressure,* which expresses the pressure exerted as the heart contracts or beats, pumping blood through the circulatory system. The bottom, or lower number, is called *diastolic pressure,* which expresses the pressure exerted when the heart is at rest between beats.

Defining high blood pressure

Many people mistakenly think that you either have hypertension or you don't. In fact, blood pressure readings span a continuum ranging all the way from *normal* to *severely elevated.* Experiencing one elevated reading does not mean that you have hypertension. Everyone's blood pressure tends to spike up in situations that produce anger, pain, fear, or high stress. For example, your blood pressure probably rises when you have a shouting match with a family member, give a speech, or interview for a new position — maybe even when you visit your friendly doctor.

Having *hypertension* means that your blood pressure is consistently elevated above the normal ranges. (It doesn't mean that you are supertense. Even the calmest, most laid-back individuals can have high blood pressure.) And knowing whether you have it is no do-it-yourself diagnosis, either. You need to have your blood pressure checked regularly, ideally as part of a regular periodic checkup. If you happen to check your blood pressure at a health fair, for example, and it's elevated, be sure to see your physician. Your physician will take your blood pressure readings on several occasions to determine whether your blood pressure is consistently elevated, and if it is, how severely elevated it is.

Identifying categories of blood pressure

For many years, until the mid-1980s, hypertension typically was defined as readings higher than 140/90 mm Hg (measured in millimeters of mercury). This rather arbitrary cutoff was chosen to define high blood pressure because the risk of cardiovascular complication becomes very significant at this point. Based on the review of the larger body of more recent research, however, a recent national medical commission formed a more sophisticated classification of high blood pressure, which you can review in Table 13-1.

Table 13-1	Classification of Blood Pressure for Adults 18 and Older*		
Category	*Systolic (mm Hg)*		*Diastolic (mm Hg)*
Normal	<120	and	<80
Prehypertension	120–139	or	80–89
Hypertension			
Stage 1	140–159	or	90–99
Stage 2	>160	or	>100

Key: < less than; > greater than, ≥ or equal to

*Reprinted from The Seventh Report of the Joint National Committee on Prevention, Detection, Evaluation and Treatment of High Blood Pressure. National Institute of Health. National Heart, Lung, and Blood Institute. National High Blood Pressure Education Program. NIH Publication No. 03-5233. May 2003.

High blood pressure

These new classifications put blood pressure into appropriate perspective. As Table 13-1 illustrates, people with a systolic blood pressure greater than 139 mm Hg or a diastolic blood pressure greater than 89 mm Hg are considered to have *hypertension*. Hypertension then is further divided into two stages of increasing severity.

Prehypertensive blood pressure

A number of large observational and clinical studies during the last decade show that people with blood pressure that is elevated from just slightly above normal to just under Stage 1 hypertension levels have at least twice the risk of developing high blood pressure. In addition, research shows that for people ages 40 to 70, the risk of heart disease doubles for every increment of 20 mm Hg in systolic blood pressure (the upper number) and 10 mm Hg in diastolic blood pressure (the bottom number) that their blood pressure goes above 115/75. As a consequence, a new classification, *prehypertension,* was established to alert individuals to this risk and to raise awareness that most people with prehypertensive blood pressure can improve their blood pressure dramatically with a few simple lifestyle modifications.

Normal blood pressure

The other important category in this new classification is *normal blood pressure.* Individuals with a systolic blood pressure of less than 120 mm Hg and a diastolic blood pressure of less than 80 mm Hg are now considered to have normal blood pressure. The new definition of normal lowers the upper limits of normal from previous definitions, because maintaining blood pressure below this level presents the lowest risk for developing heart disease, stroke, kidney disease, and other conditions associated with high blood pressure.

Low blood pressure

Is it possible to have blood pressure that's too low? Yes. But you have to have a very low blood pressure, indeed, before it becomes a problem, called *hypotension.* People who have systolic blood pressure less than 90 and diastolic pressure of less than 60 (less than 90/60 mm Hg) may actually have blood pressure that is too low. For the vast majority of people, however, the range of normal blood pressure is so great that *normal* remains an important distinction. Depending upon your individual situation, your physician may advise you that your optimal blood pressure should be well below the upper limits of normal.

Understanding the Dangers and Causes of Hypertension

Hypertension isn't called a killer for nothing. High blood pressure is a significant risk factor for developing coronary artery disease (CAD), the leading cause of death in the United States, and it's considered a significant risk for stroke, heart failure, and kidney failure. Anyone with poorly treated hypertension at least doubles his or her risk of developing all of these conditions. And remember, the higher the blood pressure, the higher the danger.

Thus, even individuals who have no symptoms when initially diagnosed with hypertension need to work hard to control blood pressure to prevent these potentially devastating complications. When you're already diagnosed with heart disease and hypertension, then controlling your blood pressure within recommended levels is perhaps the most important step you can take toward preventing or slowing the progress of your heart disease.

Determining the causes of hypertension

In the vast majority (more than 90 percent) of people with high blood pressure, physicians aren't able to determine its exact cause. In medical terms, this condition is known as _idiopathic_ hypertension. That's not to say that physicians are idiots, but that they haven't yet figured out the precise mechanisms, functions, or agents that cause hypertension. Hypertension of an undetermined cause also is termed _essential_ high blood pressure. In the same way that _idiopathic_ doesn't mean that doctors are idiots, neither does _essential_ mean that having hypertension is essential. Quite the contrary! Treating it is what _is_ essential! Look at some of the factors that appear to contribute to hypertension.

- **Salt intake:** Among the theories about what causes essential high blood pressure, most relate to problems that your kidneys appear to have with handling excess salt. Population studies show that societies in which people consume large amounts of salt (such as the United States) have a correspondingly high incidence of high blood pressure. Similarly, in cultures where salt intake is low, the incidence of high blood pressure is extremely low. Other studies show that for most people with hypertension, restricting salt intake helps lower high blood pressure.

- **Inherited predisposition:** Hypertension also appears to have a genetic component. Some people may be genetically predisposed to have high blood pressure. However, although hypertension runs in some families, these tendencies may actually result as much from shared lifestyles as they do from shared genetic backgrounds. Doctors certainly know that lifestyle factors, such as obesity (and abdominal obesity, in particular), inactivity, cigarette smoking, and high alcohol consumption all are associated with increased risk of hypertension.

- **Known conditions that cause it:** In approximately 10 percent of the people with hypertension, the specific underlying cause can be discovered. This condition is known as _secondary hypertension,_ meaning it's a secondary result of a separate primary condition. If the underlying condition can be treated and corrected, then secondary hypertension usually is corrected, too. Conditions known to cause secondary high blood pressure include

- Narrowing of the arteries that supply the kidneys

- Other diseases of kidneys

- Abnormalities in the endocrine system, such as overactive adrenal glands

- Transient conditions such as pregnancy for certain women

- Certain medications that can increase the risk of high blood pressure, such as oral contraceptives or estrogen replacement therapy following menopause

If you're diagnosed with high blood pressure, your doctor will explore any of these potential underlying causes for hypertension prior to making the diagnosis.

Checking out other risk factors

Although medical science may not know the exact mechanisms that cause essential hypertension, a number of conditions are strongly associated with increases in high blood pressure. Arresting any one of this gang of probable causes usually leads to lower blood pressure. For many people, controlling these conditions actually returns their blood pressure to normal levels.

- ✔ **Obesity:** Hypertension is most clearly associated with obesity (weighing more than 20 percent above your desirable body weight). Obesity contributes to an estimated 40 percent or more of all high blood pressure cases in the United States. Although not everyone who is overweight has high blood pressure, the association remains crystal clear.

- ✔ **Cigarette smoking:** Cigarette smoking and the use of other tobacco products increase blood pressure, both in the short term while you're smoking or chewing and in the long term, because components in the smoke or chewing tobacco, such as nicotine, cause your arteries to constrict. Childhood experiments with the nozzle on a garden hose indicate what happens when you force the same volume of liquid through a smaller opening. That higher pressure isn't a happy thing for your arteries.

- ✔ **Alcohol intake:** Drinking small to moderate amounts of alcohol (fewer than two beers, two glasses of wine, or one shot of distilled spirits) per day has been shown in a number of studies to reduce mortality from CAD. Higher consumption of alcohol (three or more alcoholic drinks per day), however, clearly is associated with increased blood pressure, not to mention an increased risk of dying from heart disease.

> ✔ **Physical inactivity:** People who are physically inactive increase their likelihood of developing high blood pressure. In one large study of more than 16,000 individuals, inactive people were 35 percent more likely to develop hypertension than were active people, regardless of whether they had a family history of high blood pressure or a personal history of being overweight.

Looking at hypertension in specific groups of people

Having high blood pressure raises some special issues for certain groups of people.

Children and adolescents

Children and adolescents who have blood pressures at levels in the top 5 percent for their age groups are considered to have elevated blood pressure. Seeking the potential underlying causes is mandatory in all children and adolescents who have high blood pressure. Because children are more likely to have secondary causes for hypertension than adults, physicians look for conditions such as abnormalities of the aorta or kidney problems that are associated with high blood pressure. In most instances, treatment for these children and adolescents involves lifestyle measures such as increased physical activity, and if the child is overweight, weight loss. Medicines are used only as a last resort and, even then, usually only for children who have extremely high blood pressure. A child or adolescent with high blood pressure needs to be treated by a pediatric cardiologist or a pediatrician who is knowledgeable in the particular demands of treating high blood pressure in young people.

The elderly

As already indicated, the older you grow, the more likely you are to have high blood pressure. And if you're older than 60 and African American, you have an even greater risk (about 15 percent higher than older people overall) of having hypertension.

Because high blood pressure is so common in older individuals, men and women alike, if you're older than 60, having your blood pressure checked frequently by your physician and paying particular attention to positive lifestyle measures, such as maintenance of normal body weight and regular physical activity, are mandatory.

African Americans

In all age groups (not only those older than 60), adults of African American descent have a higher prevalence of high blood pressure than do Americans of other ethnic groups. Furthermore, the condition appears to be more dangerous in African Americans. Compared with the general U.S. population, African Americans experience three times as much hypertension-related kidney failure, 80 percent more stroke-related deaths, and a 50 percent higher mortality rate from heart disease. African Americans also have been shown to suffer more damage to their kidneys than Caucasians at comparable levels of blood pressure.

Although the causes underlying this difference, like the underlying causes for most hypertension, remain unknown, ongoing research suggests several possibilities.

✔ **Later diagnosis and treatment:** Many African Americans may not receive treatment for high blood pressure until they've had the condition for some time and damage has occurred.

✔ **Greater sensitivity to salt:** Recent research suggests that some African Americans have a genetic trait that increases salt sensitivity and its corresponding effect on elevating blood pressure.

✔ **High salt and low potassium intake:** Many African Americans eat diets that are high in salt and low in potassium, both factors associated with elevated blood pressure.

Fortunately, research shows that when African Americans receive appropriate treatment using current therapies, their success in controlling blood pressure equals that of Caucasians receiving identical treatment. Because of the prevalence of high blood pressure and earlier onset, if you're an African American, you need to be sure to have your blood pressure checked regularly, and the childhood or teenage years are not too early.

People with diabetes mellitus

High blood pressure is much more common in individuals with diabetes than it is in the general population; moreover, it is particularly dangerous for them, because it carries a high risk of cardiovascular complications. Individuals with high blood pressure *and* diabetes are extremely susceptible to this *double trouble,* because of the increased risk of suffering damage to their kidneys, which, in turn, increases the risk of high blood pressure. For all these reasons, individuals with diabetes need to be carefully monitored for high blood pressure, and this condition needs to be treated aggressively. The latest recommendations are that people with diabetes maintain a blood pressure of less than 130/85 mm Hg.

Pregnancy

Some women develop high blood pressure during the third trimester of pregnancy. This condition is called *gestational hypertension,* and it needs to be treated cautiously by a physician who is familiar with the patient and this condition. The physician must also carefully distinguish gestational hypertension from *preeclampsia,* which is a potentially lethal condition. Fortunately, women who develop gestational hypertension have no apparent increased risk of hypertension following the pregnancy, compared with the general population.

If a pregnant woman has been diagnosed with hypertension before she becomes pregnant, or if she develops it before the 20th week of pregnancy, she is described as having *chronic hypertension.* This condition also needs to be treated by a physician experienced with treating high blood pressure during pregnancy.

The goal of treating high blood pressure during pregnancy, regardless of whether it's gestational or chronic, is lowering any health risks to the pregnant woman and the baby. For these reasons, and many others, prenatal care is important for all pregnant women.

Taking Charge of Your Blood Pressure

Controlling many of your daily habits and practices can help you prevent high blood pressure or manage existing hypertension. Taking these lifestyle measures also is an important adjunct to treatment even if you require medicines to control your blood pressure.

Managing your weight

For overweight individuals, even those who are only 15 or 20 pounds overweight, weight reduction is a highly reliable way of lowering blood pressure. Most studies indicate that you lose approximately 1 mm Hg from both your systolic and diastolic blood pressure for every two pounds that you lose. Thus, even small amounts of weight loss can make a profound difference in blood-pressure control. Individuals who lose 10 pounds can anticipate a 5 mm to 7 mm Hg reduction in their systolic and diastolic blood pressure levels. For that reason, your doctor is likely to first recommend weight reduction if you're overweight and have high blood pressure.

Getting regular physical activity

Use it (your body) and lose it (your high blood pressure). Physically active individuals reduce their risk of developing hypertension by 20 percent to 50 percent when compared with their couch potato peers. Individuals who already have hypertension can often lower their blood pressure by 5 mm Hg to 10 mm Hg simply by participating in moderately intense aerobic activity 30 to 45 minutes most days of the week. If you have hypertension, you

✔ Must conduct your physical activity at a *moderate level,* which means reducing the intensity of your exercise to a level slightly less than that recommended for individuals your age without hypertension (see Chapter 21 for more details about moderate exercise).

✔ Don't need to take your 30 to 45 minutes of physical activity all at one time but may accumulate it during the course of the day.

The benefits of regular physical activity for controlling blood pressure are added to those of weight loss.

Eating a low-sodium, heart-healthy diet

Many aspects of proper nutrition play significant roles in blood pressure control, so adopting a heart-healthy way of eating is a wise choice (see Chapter 20). Perhaps most important, however, individuals with high blood pressure need to consume a diet that is low in sodium. The American Heart Association recommends a diet that contains no more than 2 grams of sodium a day. That's equivalent to about 1 teaspoon of table salt.

The best ways to lower sodium in your diet are by

✔ Removing the saltshaker from the table

✔ Not adding extra salt to food

✔ Emphasizing fresh fruits and vegetables and grains

✔ Avoiding salty snacks and processed foods

Your doctor, often working in conjunction with a registered dietitian, can help you build a plan for eating that achieves these goals. This plan may include a role for increasing potassium in your diet. Fresh fruits and vegetables often are often high in potassium.

Avoiding tobacco use

Cigarette smoking, chewing tobacco, and other uses of tobacco have been repeatedly shown to raise blood pressure. The good news is that within a few months after quitting cigarette smoking, you'll experience a significant reduction in your blood pressure. I discuss the benefits of quitting in Chapter 23.

Limiting alcohol intake

If you consume alcoholic beverages, do so only in moderation (no more than two alcoholic drinks a day if you're a man and one if you're a woman). If having a few drinks with friends is the way you unwind at the end of the day, try some alternative ways of relaxing — join a gym or aerobics class, check out the local coffee (decaffeinated, of course) shops, or play a team sport.

Chilling out to reduce stress

If you're in a stressful environment, finding ways to reduce stress often helps lower your blood pressure. Check out the suggestions in Chapter 22.

Working with Your Doctor to Control Your Blood Pressure

If you want to succeed in combating high blood pressure, which has no immediate symptoms and lasts for many years, you need to develop a long-term partnership with your physician. Doing so typically involves three stages.

Getting a medical evaluation

The diagnosis of high blood pressure requires at least two or three different blood pressure readings on separate visits to your doctor's office, indicating that your blood pressure is consistently greater than 140/90 mm Hg.

If your blood pressure is elevated above 120/80 mm Hg to just under 140/90 mm Hg, you may have prehypertensive blood pressure (see the earlier section "Prehypertensive blood pressure"). In that case, your doctor may ask you to help in the diagnosis by monitoring your blood pressure at home. A number of excellent home monitoring devices are available that can provide accurate readings at home, and your doctor may recommend one. Don't be surprised if your blood pressure is slightly lower at home than it is at the doctor's office. This phenomenon is called the *white coat syndrome,* because a number of people get nervous in their doctor's office, and being nervous is one of the emotional states that can elevate blood pressure temporarily.

Determining treatment

The second phase in combating hypertension is treatment. Depending upon the severity of your hypertension, your physician may first ask you to make some of the lifestyle changes I discuss earlier in this chapter to help control your blood pressure. Your doctor may also prescribe medications in conjunction with these lifestyle measures to provide additional blood pressure control. I discuss more about medications in the "Using medicines to treat hypertension" section later in this chapter.

Self-monitoring

After diagnosing your high blood pressure, your doctor normally asks you to participate as a partner in your own care by

- ✔ Monitoring and keeping a log of your blood pressure.

- ✔ Following prescribed lifestyle modifications with commitment.

- ✔ Taking your medication (if it's prescribed) faithfully and as directed. Astonishingly, more than 50 percent of all medicines prescribed either are not taken at all or not taken correctly. Controlling your blood pressure is virtually impossible if you don't meticulously follow prescribed lifestyle measures and medication regimens.

- ✔ Honestly sharing with your doctor any problems or side effects you're having with either lifestyle modifications or medications. Doing so often is a crucial key to your success, because it enables you and your doctor to make necessary adjustments. Don't worry that you'll be a bother — doctors know that it can take time to fine-tune a treatment regimen to work best for you. If your doctor seems too rushed or reluctant to work with you, find one who isn't.

Selecting a home blood pressure monitor

Many brands and types of home blood pressure monitors are available. Any of the three basic types may work well for you. If you're not sure how to operate the device you select, the staff in your doctor's office will be happy to show you.

Mercury-based monitor: Known as a *sphygmo-manometer*, this device is the gold standard of monitors against which all others are measured. Your doctor's office probably uses one. It features a long glass gauge displaying a column of mercury, a cuff, and an inflator bulb. It's used with a stethoscope. Because mercury is poisonous and because these devices are a little clumsy to use, mercury monitors aren't usually recommended for home use. They do, however, give you accurate, consistent measurements during the long-term because they don't need periodic readjustment.

Electronic or digital monitor: Recent advances in the sensitivity and reliability of electronic monitoring devices have made these monitors much more accurate. Because they're easy to use, have clear displays, work with one hand, and don't require the use of a stethoscope, many people prefer them. They come in versions that have either manually or automatically inflated cuffs. Reliable digital wrist monitors also are available. *Warning:* Avoid small digital finger monitors and the like (often sold in cheap mail-order catalogs), because most of these so-called monitors are highly inaccurate and a waste of your money.

Aneroid monitors: These monitors are similar to mercury equipment, except that they have a dial-type gauge (rather than mercury), and they can get out of whack and need readjustment. These monitors have a gauge, cuff, inflator bulb, and stethoscope. If you choose one of these, you may want to make sure that the cuff has a D-ring for easy one-handed use and a self-bleeding deflation valve so that you can concentrate on measuring accurately (rather than on trying to let the air out properly).

Whatever monitor you select, be sure that you follow the manufacturer's instructions to the letter. Remember, if you need help, ask your doctor's staff for some basic instruction.

Using medicines to treat hypertension

To medicate or not to medicate? That is the question. When Hamlet raised his famous question, "To be or not to be," he was voicing a philosophical dilemma. Your physician often faces the dilemma of whether you need medication in addition to lifestyle measures. Medicines are definitely indicated whenever positive lifestyle measures haven't succeeded in adequately lowering your blood pressure. In this situation, your physician has many excellent medications to choose from.

Adding to the dilemma, different medications also work differently for different individuals. So a period of adjustment may be needed to find out just which medication or combination of medications works best for you. The latest treatment guidelines note that most individuals require two or more medications used simultaneously to reach blood pressure goals. If your doctor needs to combine several medications, they often will come from different classes.

The following three general classes of medications typically are used in controlling high blood pressure.

- **Diuretics:** The first choice of many physicians, diuretics lower blood pressure by lowering blood volume through increasing the amount of sodium and water passed through the kidneys. With regular diuretic therapy, blood pressure often falls 10 mm Hg.

- **Alpha blockers and beta blockers:** These medications inhibit various portions of the nervous system, particularly receptors called *alpha* and *beta receptors.* Inhibiting them helps lower blood pressure by slowing the heart rate and decreasing the force with which the heart pumps or by helping arteries to relax or dilate, thus lowering the pressure required to pump blood through the arteries. Among physicians, beta blockers are another popular first choice as treatment for high blood pressure.

- **Vasodilators:** These drugs act directly on the walls of the arteries and cause them to relax, thereby reducing the amount of pressure needed to pump blood through the arteries. The two major types of vasodilators in use are

  - **ACE inhibitors:** These drugs help reduce blood pressure by decreasing substances in the blood that cause vessels to constrict. The acronym ACE stands for *angiotensin converting enzyme.* Both short-acting (taken several times a day) and long-acting (typically taken once a day) ACE inhibitors are available for treatment of high blood pressure. Your physician may want to monitor kidney function and potassium levels closely when starting or increasing this medication.

  - **Calcium antagonists:** Also called *calcium channel blockers,* calcium antagonists inhibit the inward flow of calcium into cardiac and blood vessel tissues, thereby reducing the tension of the heart and the constriction of blood vessels.

- **Combination medicines:** As I mentioned in the previous section, the majority of people require two medicines to control their high blood pressure. Obtaining those medications in a combined form often is possible and makes taking them simpler. If you're taking two or more medications for hypertension, ask your doctor whether a combination medicine is right for you.

Ten tips for controlling your blood pressure for a lifetime

Because complications from high blood pressure are the result of years of increased pressure pounding on blood vessels walls, adopting a lifelong approach to controlling hypertension is important. Remember that the goal is not simply to lower blood pressure in the short-term but rather to reduce the long-term devastating complications of hypertension.

To achieve that goal, follow these ten tips:

✔ Always keep in mind that the goal of treatment is to reduce blood pressure and the complications of poorly controlled hypertension.

✔ Become knowledgeable about hypertension.

✔ Make a commitment to help your physician control your blood pressure by actively joining in a partnership to assist in your therapy.

✔ Maintain regular contact with your physician.

✔ Routinely monitor your blood pressure at home.

✔ Take your medicines the way your doctor prescribes them.

✔ Integrate medicine-taking into your daily living routines.

✔ Adopt positive lifestyle behaviors to help lower your blood pressure.

✔ Monitor side effects and report any troublesome ones to your physician.

✔ Maintain a positive attitude about achieving the goal of life-long blood pressure control.

Treating resistant hypertension

Some individuals have a condition called *resistant hypertension*. These individuals often require a combination of lifestyle measures coupled with two or three medications to control their high blood pressure. If you experience this situation, keep working closely with your physician. Blood pressure can almost always be controlled, even if you have resistant hypertension, provided that you meticulously follow the regimens that are developed in partnership with your physician.

Chapter 14

Controlling Cholesterol

Cholesterol always seems to be in the news. For a while, Americans were so obsessed with lowering blood cholesterol that other important risk factors for heart disease were almost ignored. Then the pendulum swung the other way as revisionists began underestimating the dangers of elevated cholesterol levels. The truth lies somewhere in between.

Without question, elevated blood cholesterol significantly increases — doubles, in fact — the risk of developing coronary artery disease (CAD). And in combination with other risk factors, cholesterol multiplies those risks many times over. So controlling cholesterol is vital to controlling the progression of heart disease and to lowering your risk of developing it. For most people, achieving that goal usually isn't hard: Some simple daily steps can make a great difference — even when you also must take medication and even when you already have heart disease.

Hearing Good News/Bad News about Cholesterol

The good news is that between 1960 and 1991, the average cholesterol level in the United States decreased from 220 mg/dL (milligrams per deciliter) to 205 mg/dL. This drop no doubt contributed to a 50 percent decline during the past 25 years in the incidence of death from heart disease. The bad news is that elevated blood cholesterol remains extremely common and heart disease still is the leading killer in the U.S. An estimated 32 percent of American men and 27 percent of American women have elevated blood cholesterol levels that put them at increased risk for developing heart disease. An even greater percentage of men and women older than 50 have elevated cholesterol levels, so Americans still have a long way to go.

The relationship between cholesterol levels and the risk of developing heart disease doesn't function like a light bulb — meaning either on or off. It's more like the gradual acceleration your car experiences entering a freeway. As cholesterol in the blood gradually rises to a level of about 200 mg/dL, the risk of developing heart disease also gradually increases. After your cholesterol goes above that level, the risk of heart disease and of dying from heart disease increases much more rapidly — as Figure 14-1 shows. By the time your cholesterol level reaches 250, your risk of dying from heart disease grows to more than twice that of individuals whose cholesterol levels are below 200.

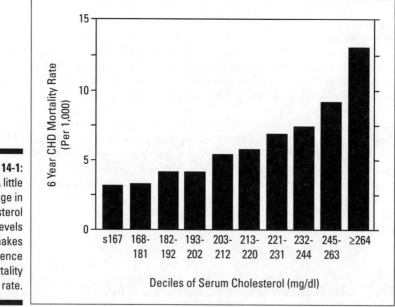

Figure 14-1:
A little change in cholesterol levels makes a difference in mortality rate.

Multiple Risk Factor Intervention Trial (MRFIT). Used with permission.

But good news! The reverse also is true. Lowering your blood cholesterol level by even a smidgen can make a positive difference. And the more you lower it, the greater the benefit. For every one point that your cholesterol drops, estimates indicate your risk of heart disease drops by 2 percent. Thus, a drop of 10 mg/dL in your cholesterol level can decrease your risk of developing heart disease by 20 percent! (Wouldn't you love returns like that on your IRA?)

Getting the Lowdown on Lipids

Cholesterol is a naturally occurring waxy substance present in human beings and all other animals. It is an important component of the body's cell walls. The body also requires cholesterol to produce many hormones (including sex hormones) and the bile acids that help it digest food. Because cholesterol plays such important biological roles, having adequate amounts of it is absolutely essential for life itself.

Humans get cholesterol from two sources. The liver manufactures a great deal, and you consume a considerable amount from animal products, such as meat, eggs, and dairy products. However, you get into trouble when you have too much cholesterol in your blood. Your level of blood cholesterol (sometimes called *serum cholesterol*) grows too high usually because you eat too much saturated fat (which encourages the liver to manufacture cholesterol) and too many foods that contain cholesterol (dietary cholesterol). Actually, you don't need to consume foods with cholesterol because your body always makes enough. In fact, in years of research, no one has ever been diagnosed with a cholesterol deficiency.

To get to where it needs to go in your body, cholesterol is carried around in your bloodstream attached to complicated structures called lipoproteins. When cholesterol levels in the blood are too high, excess cholesterol is deposited on the inside walls of the arteries in the form of *plaque,* which causes arteries to narrow. The result is the condition known as atherosclerosis, which is the basis of coronary heart disease (see Chapter 4).

Understanding lipoproteins: The good, the bad, and the ugly

And just what is a lipoprotein? A *lipoprotein* is a cross between a lipid, such as cholesterol or triglycerides, and a protein. There now, don't you know a lot more. Would it help if I told you that *lipid* comes from the Greek word for *fat?* (Yes, *fat* as in *lipo*suction.) Lipoprotein serves as the mode of transportation for cholesterol and other lipids (fats) through the bloodstream. Lipoproteins are sort of like a cruise ship steaming across the Atlantic Ocean. View the ship as the proteins and all the passengers on board (including the Family Cholesterol) as the lipids. Not a perfect analogy, but you get the point.

Lipoproteins can be separated and measured according to their weight and density. They range from very low density to high density. One particularly dangerous form is called LDL or *low-density lipoprotein. LDL* is dangerous, because it contains more fat and less protein, which makes it fairly unstable. Because it's unstable, LDL tends to fall apart and as a result easily adheres to artery walls. Because LDL cholesterol plays such a major role in forming atherosclerotic plaque, lowering LDL levels in the blood is an important goal in controlling cholesterol.

On the other hand, a beneficial type of lipoprotein called *HDL,* or *high-density lipoprotein,* can actually help protect your heart from heart disease. HDL is stable and doesn't adhere to artery walls. Instead, it actually helps carry cholesterol away from artery walls. This effect is particularly important for the coronary arteries. Keeping HDL at recommended levels helps control overall cholesterol and its potential negative effects.

When you have a checkup, your doctor may look at the results of your blood tests and say, "Well, you need to work on raising your *good cholesterol* and lowering your *bad cholesterol.*" That can be a little confusing until you realize that their names offer you a tip for keeping track of which is which. You want to keep your high-density lipoproteins (HDLs) *high* and your low-density lipoproteins (LDLs) *low.* Repeat after me: High, *high!* Low, *low!* Forgetting this mantra can result in ugly consequences for your arteries.

Tracking elevated blood triglycerides

Fats also are carried through the bloodstream in a form known as triglycerides. Although *triglycerides,* like cholesterol, are lipids, they have a different makeup. As the name suggests, these chemicals are made up of three (hence *tri*) fat molecules (fatty acids) carried through the bloodstream on a glycerol backbone. Much like cholesterol, the triglycerides are ferried around the bloodstream by joining with proteins in the form of lipoproteins. Although the link between elevated blood triglycerides and heart disease isn't as strong as the link between LDL cholesterol and heart disease, having elevated blood triglycerides nevertheless puts you at increased risk for CAD.

Defining guidelines for healthy lipid levels

Based on an analysis of a large body of research, the National Cholesterol Education Program, which represents dozens of major health organizations, defined new classifications for cholesterol and other lipids. These classifications are widely used by physicians and medical research scientists in detecting, evaluating, and treating cholesterol problems.

Table 14-1 summarizes these classifications. Measurements are expressed in milligrams (mg) of cholesterol per deciliter (dL) of blood.

Table 14-1	Classification of Cholesterol Levels
Health Risk Category	*Total Cholesterol Level*
Desirable	<200 mg/dL
Borderline high	200–239 mg/dL
High	≥240 mg/dL
	LDL Cholesterol Level
Optimal	<100 mg/dL
Near optimal/above optimal	100–129 mg/dL
Borderline high	130–159 mg/dL
High	160–189 mg/dL
Very high	≥190 mg/dL
	HDL Cholesterol Level
Low	<40 mg/dL
High	≥60 mg/dL
Optimal ratio total cholesterol to HDL	3.5:1
	Triglycerides
Normal	<150 mg/dL
Borderline high	150–199 mg/dL
High	200–499 mg/dL
Very high	≥500 mg/dL

Key: >greater than, ≥equal to or greater than, <less than

Adapted from ATP III — Third Report of the National Cholesterol Education Program (NCEP) Expert Panel on Detection, Evaluation, and Treatment of High Blood Cholesterol in Adults (Adult Treatment Panel III). Final Report. National Heart, Lung, and Blood Institute. National Institutes of Health. NIH Publication No. 02-5215. September 2002.

Lowering total cholesterol and LDL cholesterol to desirable levels and raising HDL cholesterol above the low levels and into a desirable ratio to total cholesterol can slow down, stop, or even reverse the buildup of harmful plaque in your arteries, thus lowering your risk of developing heart disease and experiencing heart attack.

Testing your cholesterol and other lipid levels

In your battle to lower cholesterol, to be at your best, you have to test. It's as simple as that. All adults (and most children) should know their respective cholesterol levels. A simple finger-stick blood test is all that's required for testing total cholesterol. You should have such a test at least every five years, or more often if your cholesterol level is elevated or if you have other risk factors for heart disease.

If the simple test shows your cholesterol level is elevated, your physician may recommend that you undergo a fasting blood test called a complete *lipid profile* or *lipid analysis* to determine your levels of LDL, HDL, and triglycerides. Physicians often include this more extensive test as part of your routine physical checkup.

If you take a simple test outside your doctor's office, perhaps at a health fair, and your cholesterol level measures 200 mg/dL or higher, be sure that you share this information with your physician so you get proper follow-up.

Decoding your cholesterol test results

Your overall cholesterol level is expressed as a number of milligrams (mg) per deciliter (dL — ⅒ of a liter) of blood: 200 mg/dL or 220 mg/dL, for example. A fasting blood test to obtain a complete lipid profile also expresses the levels of LDL and HDL as milligrams per deciliter (mg/dL). The results may also compare the level of HDL (the good guys, remember) to your total cholesterol level. This comparison is usually expressed as a ratio; for example, 3:1 or 4.5:1 means that you have one unit of HDL for every 3 or 4.5 equal units of total cholesterol. (Sometimes just the first number appears on the test report; the 1 is implied.) The most exciting thing about this arcane knowledge, however, is that you don't need even the foggiest idea of what milligrams or deciliters are to understand how to use these numbers effectively.

Equating cholesterol levels with risk of heart disease

Here are some general guidelines for interpreting what your cholesterol measurements indicate about your risk of developing heart disease or of experiencing increased complications if you already have it:

  ✔ If you don't already have existing CAD, a total cholesterol level below 200 mg/dL is considered a *desirable blood cholesterol*. But please remember that within a broad range of values, lower is better. Thus, a cholesterol level of 170 mg/dL is better than a cholesterol level of 190 mg/dL.

✔ A cholesterol level of between 200 mg/dL and 239 mg/dL is considered *borderline high blood cholesterol*. If your cholesterol is within this range, your physician will strongly recommend lifestyle modifications and perhaps medication depending on your current practices and risk factors.

✔ If your blood cholesterol level is 240 mg/dL or more, you're classified as having *high blood cholesterol*. Your physician typically will work closely with you to establish an aggressive treatment program.

✔ If your LDL cholesterol levels are above or near optimal (100 mg/dL to 129 mg/dL), most physicians will recommend using lifestyle measures that lower LDL. It's never too early to pay attention to these bad actors. In fact, treatment guidelines urge physicians to target LDL first and more aggressively in guiding patients.

✔ A low HDL cholesterol level also is considered an independent risk factor for heart disease, over and above total cholesterol and LDL levels. Individuals whose HDL is below 40 mg/dL are considered to have *low HDL cholesterol*.

✔ If your triglycerides are below 129 mg/dL, they're considered to be *optimal or near optimal*. This recommended classification, and all the other levels for triglycerides listed in Table 14-1, are new, and they may be much lower than you and perhaps even your physician are aware. The lower target ranges take into account the associations between triglycerides and other lipid and nonlipid risk factors. In addition to increasing your risk of CAD, very high levels of triglycerides may also injure the pancreas, a vital organ that is responsible for producing insulin in the body.

Treating and Managing Cholesterol Problems

Here's a riddle for you: How is cholesterol control different from spandex? When it comes to controlling cholesterol, one size definitely doesn't fit all. In determining how best to control your cholesterol, your physician takes into account not only your cholesterol level and personal history but also a number of other factors, such as your age and gender and whether you already have CAD. The intensity and components of a plan vary depending on these factors, but in all cases, treatment focuses on positive lifestyle factors, such as proper nutrition, increased physical activity, and optimal weight management.

Taking an overview of typical cholesterol treatment

By first looking at an overview of how cholesterol usually is controlled you can then find out more about some specific individual situations. Here are typical treatments for various cholesterol levels:

- ✔ **If your cholesterol level is at or below 200 mg/dL and you show neither evidence of CAD nor other major risk factors,** then no treatment is necessary. Just keep eating sensibly and staying active.

- ✔ **If your cholesterol is elevated (higher than 200 mg/dL) but your LDL is within acceptable levels and you have few other risk factors and no evidence of coronary heart disease,** then you may receive relatively less intensive therapy. Proper nutrition and increased physical activity are the primary ways to lower your cholesterol and raise your HDL levels. If your cholesterol level is very high in this scenario, your physician may also recommend medication.

- ✔ **If your cholesterol is elevated (higher than 200 mg/dL) and you have other risk factors, including elevated LDL cholesterol and/or low HDL cholesterol,** then you may undergo a moderately intensive treatment program that focuses on positive lifestyle changes, such as proper nutrition, weight management, and increased physical activities. If your cholesterol level is very high, your physician may also prescribe medication.

- ✔ **If your cholesterol is elevated (higher than 200 mg/dL) and you already have established CAD and/or are at high risk to suffer from its complications such as angina or heart attack,** then you may receive the most intensive therapy, which more than likely will include substantial lifestyle modifications and medication.

Individualizing cholesterol treatment plans

Now that you're aware of how cholesterol levels usually are controlled, here are some of the treatment plans that focus more on the individual:

- ✔ **If you have risk factors other than elevated cholesterol,** the approach that you and your physician take to help you manage elevated blood cholesterol should take into account not only your cholesterol and lipid levels but also the other risk factors you exhibit (see Chapter 3). Some risk factors such as hypertension, high LDL, low HDL, and diabetes influence therapies for elevated blood cholesterol.

✔ **If you already have CAD, diabetes, or peripheral vascular disease and may have even suffered a complication, such as angina or heart attack** (see also Chapters 4 and 5), the goal of treatment is preventing further complications. In medicine, this technique is known as *secondary prevention* and indicates that the goal is preventing second and third events, or complications, in people who already have an established problem. If you fall into this category, your physician may want to dramatically lower your LDL cholesterol, probably to below 100 mg/dL. The rationale for lowering your LDL cholesterol to this degree is that many studies show that doing so may reduce the likelihood of further complications of heart disease and may even contribute to reversing heart disease.

✔ **If you have low HDL cholesterol,** remember that you're running an independent increased risk of heart disease, over and above high levels of LDL or total cholesterol. Although not many therapeutic options are available for raising HDL, your physician may certainly recommend that you increase your physical activity, which can help raise HDL. Certain lipid-lowering medications, in particular fibric acids and niacin, also are known for raising HDL levels.

✔ **If you're a young adult, premenopausal woman, or man younger than 35,** your long-term risk of CAD increases if you have an elevated cholesterol level, but you're still considered at moderately low risk. Thus, if you exhibit no other risk factors for heart disease, your physician may recommend improved nutritional practices and weight management (if you're overweight) coupled with increased physical activity (if you're currently sedentary). Medications to lower your cholesterol may be recommended only when your cholesterol is extremely high or if you experience other significant risk factors for CAD.

✔ **If you're older,** remember that age is an independent risk factor for heart disease. The older you get, the greater your risk for developing CAD. But if you reach the age of 65, your chance of reaching the age of 80 is greater than 80 percent! Thus, prevention is important — and possible — at any age. Because many older individuals with elevated cholesterol also have other chronic illnesses, seeking the advice of your physician is particularly important, because in this situation, some of the medications for lowering cholesterol interact with medications you're taking for other chronic or acute conditions.

✔ **If you're a woman,** you may underestimate the dangers of CAD — the way all too many women do — and therefore tend to underestimate the importance of controlling cholesterol. Remember that heart disease is the leading cause of death in women — and in men. This factor is particularly true for postmenopausal women. Blood cholesterol levels among American women increase sharply around age 40 and continue to rising until more than half of women older than 55 need to lower their cholesterol levels.

Managing your cholesterol with three key lifestyle steps

How you choose to conduct your daily life in three important areas can help lower your elevated blood cholesterol. The key lifestyle decisions involve committing yourself to proper nutrition, including low fat and low cholesterol consumption, increasing physical activity, and maintaining a healthy weight.

Eating a heart-smart diet

The overall goals of providing proper nutrition to people with elevated blood cholesterol are to help them lower their cholesterol levels while maintaining a balanced and nutritionally adequate eating pattern. Guidelines for accomplishing these goals were developed by the American Heart Association (AHA) and by the National Cholesterol Education Program (NCEP) from The National Institutes of Health. As a starting point for managing your cholesterol, if your cholesterol levels are desirable or borderline, I recommend the AHA's "Eating Plan for Healthy Americans" as a starting point for managing cholesterol intake. The AHA guidelines are consistent with the Healthy Heart Diet Guide from the NCEP, but they're just a little stricter on the upper limits of overall fat consumption. Table 14-2 shares these recommendations.

Table 14-2	AHA Recommendations
AHA Eating Plan for Healthy Americans Recommendations	
Total calories should be adjusted to reach and maintain a healthy weight.	
Saturated fat intake should be 7% to 10% of total calories (or even less)	
Polyunsaturated fat intake should be up to 10% of total calories.	
Monounsaturated fat can make up to 15% of total calories.	
Total fat intake should be 30% or less of total calories.	
Dietary cholesterol intake should be less than 300 mg per day	
Sodium intake should be less than 2400 mg per day	

American Heart Association. "An Eating Plan for Healthy Americans." AHA Web site: www.americanheart.org/presenter.jhtml?identifier=1088

The principles of the Eating Plan for Healthy Americans follow the general eating patterns recommended for good health by essentially every major health organization in America. Check out Chapter 20 to find out what this approach to heart-healthy eating means in terms of real food. Even if you don't have heart disease, the principles of this diet constitute the best thinking for overall good nutrition for every adult. In reality, these eating principles also constitute proper eating for any child older than the age of 2. A somewhat higher fat intake is recommended for babies and infants younger than 2 to promote brain development.

For those of you who have high cholesterol or are at higher risk of heart disease, and for whom the eating plan in Table 14-2 is insufficient for lowering blood cholesterol below 200 mg/dL, the AHA and NCEP recommend the Therapeutic Lifestyle Changes (TLC) Diet that's part of the NCEP's program of the same name. The AHA calls the TLC Diet the next generation of the Step II Diet that previously was recommended for people in need of more aggressive changes. Because the TLC Diet is somewhat more restrictive, undertaking the plan with the advice and counsel of a registered dietitian is the best way to ensure that your nutritional needs are adequately met in your overall eating plan. Table 14-3 shows you the basic TLC Diet guidelines.

Table 14-3	TLC Diet Guidelines
TLC Diet Guidelines	
Less than 7% of the day's total calories from saturated fat	
Up to 10% of total calories from polyunsaturated fat	
Up to 20% of total calories from monounsaturated fat	
15%–35% of the day's total calories from fat	
50%–60% of total calories from primarily complex carbohydrates, particularly whole grains, fruits, and vegetables	
Dietary fiber of 20–30 grams daily, particularly soluble fiber	
Less than 200 mg of dietary cholesterol a day	
Limit sodium intake to 2400 mg a day	
Just enough calories to achieve or maintain a healthy weight and reduce your blood cholesterol.	

Adapted from ATP III — Third Report of the National Cholesterol Education Program (NCEP) Expert Panel on Detection, Evaluation, and Treatment of High Blood Cholesterol in Adults (Adult Treatment Panel III). Final Report. National Heart, Lung, and Blood Institute. National Institutes of Health. NIH Publication No. 02-5215. September 2002.

Both dietary plans recommend making dietary modifications in the context of overall lifestyle goals, such as maintaining healthy weight and getting appropriate physical activity.

Many people suffer from the misconception that food cannot be enjoyable and tasty as part of an eating plan to lower cholesterol (or control high blood pressure). The sample recipes in the Appendix at the back of this book are compatible with the Eating Plan for Healthy Americans. Several are compatible with the TLC Diet. These recipes, contributed by top American chefs, show that heart-healthy eating can be satisfying and delicious. For an entire book full of such tasty, heart-healthy recipes see *The Healthy Heart Cookbook For Dummies* (Wiley).

Getting at least 30 minutes of physical activity daily

A sedentary lifestyle, which I discuss at length in Chapter 21, is a strong and established risk factor for CAD. The good news is that increased physical activity — at least 30 minutes a day — not only lowers your overall risk for CAD, but it also helps you with cholesterol problems. Regular aerobic activity actually increases HDL cholesterol, which, in turn, is associated with decreased risk of heart disease. Even moderately intense physical activity, such as brisk walking, can raise HDL cholesterol. Of course, if you've been sedentary or already have established CAD, you need to check with your physician before starting a program of increased physical activity.

Maintaining a healthy weight

Next to proper nutritional practices, weight loss is the most important lifestyle intervention for lowering elevated cholesterol if you're overweight. Weight reduction helps lower your LDL cholesterol, lower triglycerides, and raise HDL cholesterol. People usually underestimate the benefit of weight reduction for correcting lipid problems. Even being 15 or 20 pounds over your optimal weight can contribute to elevated cholesterol levels.

Using drug treatment for high cholesterol

In some instances, managing high cholesterol requires lipid-lowering medications in addition to lifestyle measures. This requirement is of particular necessity if

- Your blood cholesterol is extremely high
- You experience other major risk factors for heart disease
- You already have established CAD

In these instances, your physician probably will recommend drug therapy, in addition to lifestyle measures, to lower elevated blood cholesterol.

Classifying medications used to treat high cholesterol

Although a bewildering variety of cholesterol medications are available, the major ones fall into one of these four categories:

- ✓ **Statins:** Numerous statin medications help lower blood cholesterol. All of them act on an enzyme that is essential for the body to produce cholesterol. The statins slow down, or inhibit, this enzyme, which is called *HMG-CoA reductase.* (Remember that tongue twister, and you'll probably be one up on your doctor!) Many studies show that these medications powerfully reduce cholesterol and lower the risk of CAD. Statin medicines are particularly useful in lowering high levels of LDL cholesterol.

- ✓ **Bile acid sequestrants:** These medications lower blood cholesterol by binding with cholesterol-containing bile acids in the intestines from which they're eliminated in the stool. Bile acid sequestrants have a long history of safe and effective use for lowering blood cholesterol. These medications are particularly valuable if you have elevated LDL cholesterol.

- ✓ **Fibric acids:** Fibric acids are particularly effective in lowering triglycerides, and they've demonstrated the ability to modestly lower LDL cholesterol. Fibric acids are particularly appropriate if you have high triglyceride levels and elevated LDL cholesterol. Tests also show that some of these medications raise HDL cholesterol — the good guys.

- ✓ **Nicotinic acid:** Nicotinic acid, which is a form of the B vitamin called niacin, is effective in lowering triglycerides and total blood cholesterol and in raising HDL cholesterol. Despite these benefits, some people may have difficulty tolerating this medication because of its side effects, which include itching and flushing of the skin and gastrointestinal distress.

  Although niacin is inexpensive and available over the counter, never self-medicate for cholesterol control, because a physician must monitor you for major dangerous side effects.

Considering the risks of estrogen replacement therapy as cholesterol therapy

Although numerous studies through the years showed that estrogen may lower LDL cholesterol and raise HDL cholesterol, a recent Hysterectomy Educational Resources & Services (HERS) Foundation study indicates that starting estrogen replacement therapy (ERT) isn't advisable for women with established CAD. In addition, the estrogen-plus-progestin part of the Women's Health Initiative (WHI) study, which was designed to examine the effectiveness of this type of hormone replacement therapy in preventing CAD in postmenopausal women who did not have it, was terminated early because health risks outweighed the benefits. Because other clinically proven medications and therapies effectively lower cholesterol (and treat osteoporosis — another potential benefit of ERT), a number of health organizations now recommend ERT only for short-term relief of the symptoms of menopause. Because of the continuing controversy surrounding ERT, fully discussing of the pros and cons of this approach for treating menopause symptoms with your physician is essential.

Following up after beginning drug therapy

If your physician starts you on medication to help lower cholesterol, having your cholesterol level tested in four to six weeks after beginning the therapy is important. If adequate blood cholesterol lowering isn't achieved, increasing the dosage or adding a second medication may be necessary. Remember, lipid-lowering medications should always be used in conjunction with positive lifestyle measures, such as proper nutrition, increased physical activity, and weight management — if you're overweight.

Regarding Special Issues in Controlling Cholesterol

Addressing special issues is an important part of you and your physician working together to lower blood cholesterol. Other health conditions you may have can influence the therapies your doctor recommends for lowering your cholesterol.

Lowering triglyceride levels

Many steps that you take in your daily life can effectively help lower blood triglycerides, including increasing your physical activity, reducing your weight if you're overweight, and restricting alcohol and simple sugars in the diet. (Is this beginning to sound familiar?) If your triglyceride levels are elevated in addition to cholesterol, various medications, in particular the fibric acids and nicotinic acid may be added to lifestyle measures to help control high triglycerides and high LDL.

Delivering a double whammy — high blood cholesterol and hypertension

Elevated blood cholesterol and elevated blood pressure (hypertension) are common afflictions in the U.S. Unfortunately, they frequently occur in tandem, and that spells double trouble because risk factors for heart disease do not add up — they multiply. For example, having elevated blood cholesterol and hypertension quadruples your risk of developing heart disease. Unfortunately, high cholesterol and high blood pressure occur together in 40 percent to 50 percent of people who initially were diagnosed with one or the other condition. This deadly combination is particularly common in overweight individuals.

If you have elevated cholesterol and high blood pressure, you must work with your physician to simultaneously lower both conditions. Controlling the combination of high blood pressure and elevated cholesterol represents a real challenge, because some of the medications used to treat one of the problems may react negatively with the other. Once again, the first line of treatment if you're overweight is weight reduction. Other lifestyle measures, such as proper nutrition, including the principles espoused in the Eating Plan for Healthy Americans, and increased physical activity can simultaneously lower elevated blood pressure and blood cholesterol. (For more information about treating hypertension, see Chapter 13.)

Multiplying trouble — elevated blood cholesterol accompanied by diabetes

Besides hypertension, another dangerous condition frequently associated with elevated blood cholesterol is Type 2 diabetes (also called *adult-onset diabetes* or *noninsulin dependent diabetes*). The lipid problems that accompany diabetes typically are elevated blood triglycerides, slightly elevated LDL cholesterol, and low HDL cholesterol.

Because Type 2 diabetes is a clear and strong independent risk factor for developing CAD, people with diabetes need to pay particular attention to having their blood lipids checked frequently. If lipid abnormalities are present and you have diabetes, you'll need aggressive treatment to correct these problems.

Similarly, a common association exists between Type 2 diabetes and obesity. Although not all diabetics are obese, more than 80 percent of all Type 2 diabetics are overweight. If you have Type 2 diabetes and you're overweight, the first and most important line of defense is losing weight.

Noting other conditions associated with cholesterol

Other medical conditions that may cause blood-lipid abnormalities include certain diseases of the kidney and liver and low thyroid levels. If you have any of these conditions, important steps to take include frequently checking your blood cholesterol and other lipid levels and discussing these issues in detail with your physician.

Considering severe and/or hereditary forms of elevated blood cholesterol

Approximately 1 percent to 2 percent of the populace of the U.S. has an inherited tendency for severely elevated blood cholesterol. Their respective conditions typically are the result of genetic traits that affect how their bodies handle cholesterol. The best advice: If any member of your family has a severely elevated cholesterol level, you and all your family members need to consult with your physicians, be screened, and receive the proper therapy, if you have one of these genetic conditions.

Chapter 15

Understanding Drug and Medical Treatments for Heart Disease

*I*f you've been diagnosed with any form of heart disease, your physician has at his or her disposal a wide variety of treatment options. Depending upon the type and severity of your heart problem and any coexisting medical conditions you may have, these options range from simple lifestyle modifications and drug therapy to complex surgery. In this chapter, I provide an overview of the medical, lifestyle, and drug treatment options that don't require surgery or other invasive procedures (which I discuss next in Chapter 16). To make it easy to follow the discussion, I group these treatment types as

✔ Emergency procedures

✔ Lifestyle modifications

✔ Drug therapies

Saving Lives with Emergency Medical Procedures

Two common emergency procedures that are used when you experience a sudden stoppage of the heart or rhythm problems are cardiopulmonary resuscitation and defibrillation. For people with heart disease, these emergency treatments can be lifesavers, but for many who have undiagnosed heart disease, these emergency procedures may be the first treatment they receive. The latter is a double-edged sword — fortunate because CPR and defibrillation save lives, yet unfortunate because knowing when you have cardiac risk factors (see Chapter 3) and getting early diagnosis of heart disease lead to better outcomes.

Cardiopulmonary resuscitation (CPR)

Cardiopulmonary resuscitation, commonly called CPR, is required when you experience sudden heart stoppage. CPR techniques were introduced approximately 25 to 30 years ago and have evolved since then.

The two main branches of CPR are

- Basic cardiac life support (BCLS)
- Advanced cardiac life support (ACLS)

Although ACLS requires training in skills and equipment found in an ambulance or hospital setting, virtually anyone can discover how to administer BCLS. Studies show that BCLS procedures can be lifesaving.

If a family member has serious heart disease, you need to learn the **ABCs** of CPR:

- Establishing an adequate **airway**
- Helping the individual **breathe**
- Establishing **circulation** by putting pressure on the chest

Courses in BCLS techniques are available in virtually every major metropolitan area in the United States. You can obtain information from the American Red Cross, a local branch of The American Heart Association, or your local health-care institution. Prompt administration of BCLS can be lifesaving. I strongly urge you to learn these techniques.

Defibrillation

Everyone who's ever watched a doctor show on TV has seen the defibrillation equipment's paddles whipped out and applied to some poor soul on the gurney. What screenwriter or director can resist such drama? And in truth, regardless of how exaggerated the TV scenarios actually are, something pretty dramatic is going on in the heart of anyone who needs the emergency procedure known as *defibrillation*.

The heart depends on a system of electrical impulses to maintain its rhythm and contract properly. Nothing good happens when this electrical system goes awry. At worst, rather than contracting, the heart simply quivers, or *fibrillates* (in cardiology this problem is called *fibrillation*). Because a heart that's experiencing ventricular fibrillation generates no blood flow and quickly leads to death, emergency action is required. Using those paddles you're so familiar with and an adjustable source of electricity, an electrical current is directed to the heart in an attempt to jumpstart it.

After CPR, the American Heart Association rates access to early defibrillation as vital to the chances of survival for a victim of sudden cardiac arrest (sudden ventricular fibrillation). The continuing development and increased availability of *automated external defibrillators* (AEDs), which weigh only a few pounds, use long-lasting batteries, and can be operated by lay people with some basic training (such as firefighters, police, flight attendants, safety officers, sports trainers) are daily proving the value of this lifesaving procedure.

Making Positive Lifestyle Modifications

Thousands of research studies have proved that taking certain positive steps in your daily lifestyle not only lower your risk of developing heart disease but also provide powerful treatment options to help you effectively manage coronary artery disease (CAD). Appropriate lifestyle modifications, often in combination with appropriate drug therapy, may prevent or lessen the need for invasive, complicated cardiovascular procedures. I've advocated this approach to good health, which I like to call lifestyle medicine, for a long time.

Lifestyle medicine is about those daily habits and practices that clearly are proven to lower your risk of heart disease. These measures help put you in control of your life, giving you that feeling of autonomy that so many people with heart disease desire. Four of these lifestyle measures are so important that I've devoted three chapters (Chapters 20–22) to showing you why and how to achieve their benefits.

Following a sound nutrition plan

Eating a diet that follows heart-healthy guidelines can help you fight and even reverse heart disease and control contributing risk factors such as high cholesterol and other lipid levels, high blood pressure, and emerging markers of CAD, such as homocysteine or C-reactive protein. Such a diet is rich in fruits, vegetables, whole grains, and fiber; low in saturated fat; and just right in calories to maintain a healthy weight. The best plan also is full of pleasures and conveniences. Chapter 20 presents simple guidelines to help you achieve these goals.

Maintaining a healthy weight

Being even 10 or 15 pounds more than your optimal weight can put you at greater risk of developing heart disease and such contributing and coexisting conditions as high blood pressure, high cholesterol levels, and diabetes. Chapter 20 provides tips and techniques for helping you lose weight and maintain a healthy weight by using a sound nutrition plan.

Getting regular physical activity

Being a couch potato isn't healthy for you or the couch (chronic spring and upholstery fatigue syndrome, don't you know). For most people who have heart disease, accumulating regular, moderate physical activity as directed by their physicians can improve blood pressure, cholesterol levels, and heart function, and can combat atherosclerosis. Regular physical activity also provides crucial support for maintaining a healthy weight. Chapter 21 discusses the essential elements of a heart-healthy physical activity plan.

Reducing stress using the power of mind/body connections

A growing body of research identifies stress as one of the factors that contribute to the injury and inflammation of the coronary arteries that trigger the beginnings of heart disease and contribute to its continued progression. Stress also exacerbates the problems of heart disease in other ways. Fortunately, using simple mind/body techniques such as visualization, relaxation, biofeedback, and other natural methods of stress reduction can clearly lower your risk of heart disease. I discuss the benefits and methods for reducing stress in Chapter 22.

Taking an Overview of Drug Therapies

Thanks to extensive, ongoing pharmacological research, physicians have a wide, ever growing array of drugs to treat the various manifestations of heart disease and the many health conditions (high blood pressure and high cholesterol included) that contribute to heart disease. Although I discuss drug therapy as part of the chapters devoted to specific conditions (such as angina, heart attack, arrhythmias, and heart failure), here I present a brief overview of the different types of drugs. Why? As I discuss in Chapter 3, the contributing risk factors and conditions for heart disease rarely occur singly. Most people with heart disease have a combination of contributing conditions or associated problems that require physicians to draw from a number of drugs to create an optimal treatment plan. For that reason, you may want to be able to review the major categories of drugs used in treating various manifestations of heart disease.

Use the following quick reference (which lists drug types in alphabetical order) to find out more.

- **Antiarrhythmics:** Approximately 30 to 40 medications are in four classes that your doctor can use to treat specific arrhythmias. For example, various medicines exist to help slow or increase heartbeat or to stabilize heart rhythm. Specific problems and some individuals may require complex combinations of antiarrhymthmic drugs, which may also need to work in concert with other heart medications.

- **Antibiotics:** Bacterial infections related to the heart and cardiovascular system, such as endocarditis, bacterial pericarditis, or rheumatic fever, require treatment with appropriate antibiotics. Individuals with heart valve conditions or replacements often must take antibiotics before dental work to protect them against bacterial infection.

- **Anticoagulants (blood thinners):** These drugs aid in preventing and treating the formation of blood clots associated with coronary artery disease and other manifestations of cardiovascular disease where clots may be a problem, such as heart attack, atrial fibrillation, stroke, peripheral vascular disease, deep vein thrombosis, or valve problems. Your doctor closely monitors your use of anticoagulants for the effectiveness of the dosage and potential problems with excessive bleeding.

- **Antidepressants:** Moderate to severe depression often occurs after you experience a heart attack or other severe heart event. In these cases, the physician may prescribe an appropriate antidepressant.

- **Anti-inflammatories:** Anti-inflammatory drugs such as aspirin (see "Aspirin" later in this list) may be prescribed to help prevent or slow the development of CAD. Other anti-inflammatories are useful for the treatment of certain heart conditions such as pericarditis (see Chapter 9).

- **Antiplatelets (platelet receptor inhibitors):** Antiplatelet medicines block the ability of platelets to contribute to clot formation. They often are used in conjunction with aspirin and/or anticoagulants, and some of them are given intravenously. Your physician may prescribe them as part of prevention or treatment for unstable angina, heart attack, stroke, or pulmonary embolism.

✔ **Aspirin:** One of the oldest medicines in the pharmacopoeia, aspirin still is one of the best and truly is a wonder drug. Because it makes platelets less sticky, aspirin clearly has been shown to lower the risk of subsequent cardiac problems for people who have underlying CAD. Doctors typically prescribe aspirin (81 to 350 mg daily) as a preventive treatment for atherosclerosis, heart attack, and stroke. Because enteric-coated aspirin appears safer to the gastrointestinal tract, cardiologists often prescribe it for individuals who need to take aspirin every day.

✔ **Beta blockers:** These drugs work through the sympathetic nervous system (see Chapter 2) to slow heart rate, decrease the force with which the heart pumps, and help the arteries relax (dilate). For these reasons, beta blockers are a primary treatment for high blood pressure. They are also useful in the treatment of stable angina and certain arrhythmias and may be valuable in treating heart failure in certain people.

✔ **Bile acid sequestrants:** Bile acid is produced when your body metabolizes cholesterol. These medicines help lower levels of blood cholesterol by combining with cholesterol-containing bile acid in the intestines and thus eliminating it from the body. They're particularly useful in lowering LDL cholesterol (the bad guys).

✔ **Digitalis (digoxin):** Because this drug increases the force of heart contractions but also slows the heart rate, it is useful in treating such disorders as heart failure and certain arrhythmias, particularly atrial fibrillation.

✔ **Diuretics:** Sometimes called "water pills," these medicines reduce fluid outside the cells in the body, passing the fluid through the kidneys and evacuating it as urine. Recent research confirms that diuretics are among the most effective and economical treatments for high blood pressure. Diuretics also are useful in treating the edema (swelling) associated with heart failure.

✔ **Fibric acids:** These drugs, also called *fibrates*, lower triglyerides and help raise HDL cholesterol (the good guys).

✔ **Inotropes:** These intravenous medicines are given to increase the heart's pumping ability. They're useful in heart failure and certain cardiomyopathies.

✔ **Nicotinic acid (niacin):** This medicine, a form of B vitamin, is effective in lowering triglycerides and total cholesterol while raising HDL cholesterol. Some individuals, however, find the itching and skin-flushing side effects it often produces difficult to tolerate.

✔ **Nitrates (nitroglycerin):** These medicines are a type of vasodilator (see "vasodilators" later in this list) that relaxes the smooth muscles in the blood vessels and heart, lowering pressure on blood vessel walls and increasing blood flow. They're useful for preventing and relieving the chest pain of angina and for treating heart failure. They also may be used as part of the treatment in acute heart attack.

✔ **Statins:** These drugs, which are known as HMG-CoA reductase inhibitors, help lower cholesterol by blocking a substance used by the liver to produce cholesterol. Because they've proved so effective, statins typically are the first-choice drug therapy for reducing cholesterol levels.

✔ **Vasodilators:** These medicines relax the blood vessels, lessening pressure on the vessel walls and allowing greater blood flow. As a consequence, they are a primary treatment for high blood pressure and are useful for treating heart failure and other conditions. Three major vasodilators are

- **ACE inhibitors:** These medicines dilate blood vessels by decreasing angiotensin-converting enzymes in the blood, which cause the vessels to constrict.

- **Angiotensin receptor blockers (ARBs):** These medicines are particularly useful for patients who can't tolerate ACE inhibitors because of side effects such as cough.

- **Calcium antagonists:** Also called *calcium channel blockers,* these medicines promote more relaxed muscles in blood vessels by blocking the entry of constriction-causing calcium into muscle cells.

Chapter 16

Treating Heart Disease with Invasive and Surgical Procedures

*A*lthough many people with heart disease manage their conditions with lifestyle modifications and drug therapy, many other problems ranging from blocked coronary arteries to heart valve failures require minimally invasive medical procedures or surgery to restore higher heart function and quality of life for the patient. In this chapter, I discuss medical and surgical procedures commonly used to treat rhythm problems, atherosclerotic narrowing and blockage of coronary arteries, and heart valve problems.

Treating Rhythm Problems with the Electric Company

Because the complex electrical impulses that control the heart's rhythm and contraction are so critical, a whole branch of cardiology has grown to detect rhythm abnormalities and correct underlying electrical problems in the heart. In addition to some of the diagnostic tests that I discuss in Chapter 11, here are the most commonly used medical or surgical electrical procedures involving the heart:

- ✔ **Cardioversion:** This procedure applies a small amount of electrical current to the heart, using the same equipment that is used for defibrillation. Although the procedure is not invasive, for clarity I've grouped it with the rest of the electric company. Cardioversion can be used to treat certain rhythm abnormalities, such as

  - Irregular beating of the heart's atria, or booster pumps *(atrial fibrillation)*

  - A rapid heartbeat originating in the booster pumps *(atrial tachycardia)*

  - A rapid heartbeat originating in the ventricles *(ventricular tachycardia)*

- ✔ **Automatic implantable cardiac defibrillators (ICD):** Thanks to technological advances, tiny defibrillators about the size of a pacemaker can be implanted in the chest wall. Cardiologists increasingly are using these devices in individuals with serious arrhythmias who have survived episodes of sudden cardiac death or who are at high risk of cardiac collapse because of heart failure. The device monitors heart rhythms and automatically delivers an appropriate shock as necessary to restore proper rhythms.

- ✔ **Pacemakers:** These devices are used, either temporarily or permanently, to speed up a heart that is beating too slowly, a condition called *bradycardia* (*brady* = slow; *cardia* = heartbeat). Pacemakers actually *pace* the heartbeat by delivering electrical impulses that are very similar to the heart's own electrical system. The typical pacemaker employed now has one electrical beat that goes into the atrium, and one that goes into the ventricle. These *A-V pacemakers* are powered by batteries that can last for many years.

  Pacemakers typically are placed in the front of the chest using a minor surgical procedure to create a pocket under the skin. The electrodes then are threaded into the right atrium or ventricle or into both, depending upon the type of pacemaker.

- ✔ **Cardiac electrophysiology:** As the most -advanced form of electrical work on the heart, electrophysiology takes place in specialized laboratories that resemble heart catheterization labs. Specialized electrical catheters are placed into various portions of the heart, where either monitoring or corrective electrical work can be performed either to diagnose or correct rhythm problems or other electrical abnormalities. For example, to treat chronic tachycardia in carefully selected patients, the electrophysiologist may perform a procedure known as *ablation,* in which heat from catheter-delivered radio frequency energy is used precisely to destroy the tiny, selected parts of the heart's electrical system that are causing the tachycardia. Because they're so specialized, electrophysiology procedures typically are performed in large hospital centers.

Understanding Percutaneous Coronary Interventions (PCIs)

When atherosclerosis (CAD) severely narrows or blocks any of the major coronary arteries, threatening to cause a heart attack, *percutaneous coronary interventions* or *PCIs* often are used to relieve the problem. That fancy word *percutaneous* simply means that the cardiologist performs the procedure through the skin. (Don't you love medspeak?) Most such procedures use a catheter that is inserted into the blocked vessel. A *fluoroscope,* which delivers real-time X-ray pictures of the vessel and catheter movements to a screen, enables the cardiologist and medical-care team to view exactly what's happening.

PCIs typically take place in cardiac catheterization labs. Patient preparation and recovery are similar for most procedures. Before the procedure, patients usually receive a sedative to relax them, anticoagulants to prevent potentially dangerous blood clots forming around the catheter or instruments during the procedure, and other medications as needed. Local anesthesia numbs the area where the catheter is inserted, usually in the femoral artery in the upper thigh but sometimes in the arm. After the procedure is finished, the patient remains in recovery until the catheter sheath is removed from the insertion site and there's no chance of bleeding or complication at that site. Patients may then either remain in hospital or go home the same day, depending on the individual patient's condition, the nature of the procedure, and the technique used for ensuring that the catheter insertion site in the artery won't bleed. If you need one of the following PCI procedures, your doctor gives you complete instructions.

Opening blocked arteries with coronary angioplasty

Coronary angioplasty, also called *balloon angioplasty,* is a minimally invasive procedure that can quickly restore or improve blood flow through blocked arteries in patients for whom the procedure is appropriate. More than a half million patients benefit from angioplasty every year. Its formal name, which you may hear from your cardiologist or find in patient information, is *percutaneous transluminal coronary angioplasty* (PTCA).

Using the technique of heart catheterization, the cardiologist moves a specialized catheter equipped with a high-pressure balloon (on its tip) into the narrowed or blocked coronary artery or arteries. Once the catheter enters the narrowed section of the artery, the balloon is inflated. The inflated balloon stretches the artery and literally squashes the plaque up against the side of the blood vessel (see Figure 16-1). This procedure opens up the artery, enabling greater blood flow.

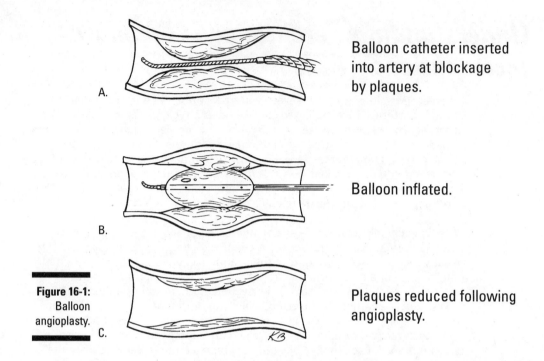

A.

Balloon catheter inserted into artery at blockage by plaques.

B.

Balloon inflated.

Figure 16-1:
Balloon angioplasty.

C.

Plaques reduced following angioplasty.

One drawback of conventional angioplasty is that in 25 percent to 40 percent of cases, the narrowing recurs in the artery, an event called *restenosis.* When that happens, another angioplasty, often including the insertion of a *stent* (a device that supports the expanded wall of the blood artery), or even bypass surgery may be necessary.

Holding arteries open with coronary stenting

In certain cases of narrowed coronary arteries in which the narrowing process appears likely to recur, the cardiologist may place a device called a stent in the area where the angioplasty has occurred. These mechanical devices look a little like coiled springs and are designed to hold blood vessels open. Stenting may take place during the first angioplasty to prevent recurrence of the narrowing or during a second angioplasty to reopen the narrowing.

Stents significantly lessen the chance that the narrowing will recur, but they don't completely prevent it. Using specialized stents called *drug-eluting stents,* which incorporate a time-release drug, can provide additional protection against renarrowing for some patients.

Another new technique that cardiologists may consider using for individuals who have experienced a renarrowing or blockage of a stented artery is *coronary brachytherapy*. This procedure uses a catheter placed inside the artery to deliver a small dose of beta or gamma radiation directly to the artery lining where the blockage is located. Although the procedure appears beneficial in the short-term, the long-term effectiveness of the procedure and the long-term effect of the radiation are not yet known because the procedure still is so new.

Removing blockages with coronary atherectomy

Coronary atherectomy may be the procedure of choice when the fatty plaque blocking the artery is very hard. In this procedure, a catheter tipped with a tiny metal cone equipped with cutting edges is used to shave away the plaque from the artery walls in a process similar to Roto-Rootering. (One more reason why invasive cardiologists are called plumbers.) The loosened plaque particles then are sucked through holes in the catheter tip and removed from the blood vessel.

Removing blockages with laser angioplasty

Laser angioplasty is similar to an atherectomy in that it also removes the plaque narrowing the artery. In this procedure a laser on the end of the catheter is used to incinerate the fatty plaque deposits.

Using angioplasty immediately after a heart attack

In certain cases immediately after an individual has had a heart attack and where the conditions are appropriate, the cardiologist may use one of the forms of angioplasty I've just discussed to remove the clot (thrombus) that caused the heart attack and/or to widen the blocked artery. The objective is restoring blood flow to the damaged part of the heart muscle as quickly as possible and thus preserving as much function as possible. This procedure can be lifesaving in some cases.

Looking at Coronary Bypass Surgery

Certain problems with severely blocked arteries may require coronary bypass surgery. In addition to conventional *coronary artery bypass grafting* (CABG — often pronounced "cabbage" in the lingo of physicians), recent research has developed several types of less invasive coronary bypass surgery that, although still in the experimental stage, nevertheless appear to offer equally effective results and shorter recovery times for selected individuals. Such surgery is performed by cardiac surgeons, who train first as general surgeons and then specialize in cardiac surgery. Although they belong to different specialties, cardiologists and cardiac surgeons work closely together. Here's a look at the "gold standard" CABG and new less -invasive bypass surgical procedures.

Understanding coronary artery bypass grafting

In coronary artery bypass grafting, a piece of vein from the leg or artery from the chest is used to bypass the blockage in a coronary artery and restore blood flow.

In the conventional form of CABG, an incision is made through the breastbone (sternum) and the chest is opened to reach the heart (hence the term *open heart surgery*). At the same time, a donor vein for the bypass graft is surgically removed (*harvested,* a surgeon would say) from the leg. In most cases, the patient also is placed on a heart-lung machine (or pump oxygenator) that takes over for the heart, which then is stopped for the surgery. The surgeon attaches one end of the bypass vein to the aorta and the other end to the blocked coronary artery below the blockage (or *occlusion*), as shown in Figure 16-2. When all the grafts to be performed are complete, the patient is removed from the heart-lung machine, and the heart is restarted. The breastbone is rejoined using surgical wires that remain permanently in place after stabilizing the breastbone and aiding in its healing. After the surgery is complete, CABG patients are carefully monitored in the Intensive Cardiac Care Unit (ICCU).

Instead of or in addition to using donor veins for the bypass, the surgeon may use a mammary artery from the chest. In this case, just one end of the graft artery is brought over and attached to the coronary artery below the blockage, and blood then flows from the mammary artery to the coronary artery.

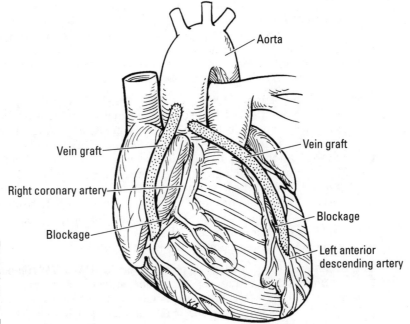

Aorta

Vein graft

Vein graft

Right coronary artery

Blockage

Blockage

Left anterior descending artery

Figure 16-2:
Heart bypass with two grafts.

Bypassing blocked coronary arteries with less invasive surgery

Conventional bypass surgery is major surgery. It's about as *major* as surgery can get. The breastbone must be split, the heart stopped, and the patient's life supported by a heart-lung machine for several hours. This surgery has a highly successful track record, but its risks and complexity offer potential for complications for many patients. Full recovery also takes about three to six months for most patients. As a result, cardiac surgeons and specialists constantly are working to develop surgical techniques that are less difficult and less risky but still produce quality outcomes for patients.

Currently, three promising, less-invasive procedures are being used in selected, appropriate cases. They are

✔ **Minimally Invasive Direct Coronary Artery Bypass (MIDCAB):** Unlike conventional CABG, in which the breastbone is split to open the chest and provide access to the heart, in MIDCAB, the cardiac surgeon works with special instruments through a small keyhole incision in the chest wall that's about 2.5 inches to 4 inches (6 cm to 10 cm) across. As part of the incision, a tiny piece of costal cartilage on the front of a rib is removed to provide access. The surgeon may or may not place the patient on a heart-lung machine, depending on individual conditions and needs. At this time, MIDCAB is suitable only for individuals whose blockages are in the left anterior descending artery on the front of the heart and who need only one or two bypasses.

✔ **Off-Pump Coronary Artery Bypass (OPCAB):** This technique has grown quickly in popularity because of increasingly sophisticated technology that enables surgeons to stabilize a beating heart to safely perform surgery on it. To perform OPCAB, the surgeon makes the same type and size incision through the breastbone as for conventional bypass surgery. Then, instead of placing the patient on a heart-lung machine, the surgeon uses a stabilizing device that holds still small sections of the heart where the surgeon is working while allowing the heart to keep beating. Benefits from OPCAB include decreased blood transfusions, decreased risk of stroke, and fewer problems with lungs, kidneys, and mental clarity, in addition to quicker recovery times.

✔ **Robot-Assisted Coronary Artery Bypass (RACAB):** Welcome to the 21st century! In this cutting-edge technique, surgeons don't perform surgery in the traditional "hands on" or "hands in" sense but manipulate a robotic device as they watch the surgical field on a video screen. The technique enables surgeons to perform precise, minimally invasive heart surgery. Researchers envision a day when surgeons may be able to perform surgery without setting foot in the same room as the patient — your RACAB procedure in Phoenix could be performed by a surgeon in Toronto! At present, RACAB is available in only a few medical centers where research continues.

Exploring Heart Valve Surgery

As I discuss in Chapter 9, injury or disease may cause heart valves to malfunction in two basic ways.

✔ **Stenosis:** Constricting or narrowing so that they do not let enough blood flow through

✔ **Regurgitation:** Leaking as the result of defects that prevent them from closing properly

Manifestations of both problems may require medical or surgical repair. Severe malfunctions may require valve replacement.

Opening narrowed valves with valvuloplasty

In *percutaneous balloon valvuloplasty,* the cardiologist inserts a catheter tipped with a high-pressure balloon through a blood vessel into the heart. After positioning the balloon in the narrowed valve, the cardiologist inflates the balloon to stretch the constricted valve. The likelihood of the valve reconstricting is about 50 percent, so this procedure is used most commonly for individuals who have only mild or moderate valve narrowing or who cannot tolerate open-heart surgery.

Repairing heart valves with surgery

Both narrowed and leaking heart valves may be repaired using open-heart surgery and the heart-lung machine. In such a procedure, the surgeon cuts into the valve to surgically remodel its structures, enabling them to function properly. The restorative results of such surgery usually are long-lasting.

Current research in valve surgery is developing minimally invasive techniques and specially designed surgical instruments (some of which use fiber optics) that will lower surgical risk and reduce recovery times.

Replacing defective heart valves

When any of the four cardiac valves becomes so damaged that it cannot function properly and cannot be repaired surgically, the damaged valve needs to be replaced with one of the following types of *prosthetic* valves.

- **Mechanical valves,** which are constructed from metal and/or other synthetic materials
- **Natural valves,** which make use of human or animal tissue and come in three types:
    - **Xenograph,** a specially cultured porcine valve from a pig or bovine valve from a cow
    - **Autograph,** a valve shaped from the patient's own tissue
    - **Homograph,** a human valve from a cadaver donor

Each of these different valves has particular advantages and disadvantages. Surgeons always discuss the pros and cons of each type of valve with their patients. As in coronary artery bypass surgery, valve repair or replacement requires open-heart surgery and the use of a heart-lung machine.

Considering Other Forms of Cardiac Surgery

Cardiac surgeons also perform operations on other aspects of the heart, including many of the conditions that I discuss in Chapter 9. In addition, cardiac surgeons may perform surgery on other structures in the chest, including removing cardiac tumors, repairing congenital heart disease, and performing various pieces of surgery on the lungs.

Chapter 17

Evaluating Alternative Therapies: Are They for You?

*Y*ou know by now that I believe you can do many things in your daily life to enhance your short- and long-term quality of life. But where do alternative therapies fit in?

Let me say right from the beginning that Western medicine doesn't have all the answers. A number of aspects of alternative therapy, a number of behaviors, and a number of products that fall under the rubric of alternative or complementary medicine can be beneficial. But because "alternative" can be used to cover so many areas, the old warning of caveat emptor — let the buyer beware — certainly applies here. However, if you're careful and use *proven* alternative-medicine techniques judiciously and in combination with the many benefits of modern Western cardiovascular medicine, you can derive important benefits without taking unnecessary risks.

In this chapter, I look at some alternative or complementary therapies that have been proven to be beneficial in the fight against heart disease. I also discuss how to judge which techniques are questionable or even pure baloney.

Defining Alternative Medicine

A number of different definitions have been offered for alternative medicine. In fact, the definition changed quite a bit during the last decade as more and more medical researchers began conducting well-designed, rigorous scientific studies to test the more promising alternative therapies. In a sense, perhaps the broadest definition defines this type of medicine by what it is *not*.

Alternative medicine is, in essence, an alternative to traditional Western medicine. It has come to include a variety of behavioral techniques, such as relaxation methods or meditation and other spiritual techniques, in addition to a number of different clinical approaches, such as chiropractic, massage, and herbal remedies. As a practical matter, it has come to include both *mind therapy* (behavioral) and *body therapy* (clinical). Mind therapies include mental imagery, hypnosis, relaxation, and so on. Body therapies include not only chiropractic but also acupuncture and herbal treatments.

Recognizing the Difference between the Placebo Effect and Proof

Emotions tend to run pretty high when people talk about alternative medicine. Some people believe that the techniques of alternative medicine have made enormous differences in their lives. However, many physicians point out that few of these techniques have been subjected to rigorous scientific testing, so little scientific evidence is available about whether many of these techniques are clinically effective.

Finding research on alternative therapies

Finding and understanding scientific information about various alternative therapies is a challenge, but the National Center for Complementary & Alternative Medicine (NCCAM), which is a branch of the National Institutes of Health, provides a number of excellent online resources, including links to Complementary and Alternative Medicine on PubMed and other databases, and tips on how you can conduct searches of alternative medicine subjects.

You can consult the NCCAM Web site at nccam.nih.gov, or call its consumer clearinghouse at 888-644-6226.

In a sense, both positions are right. Thanks to the complex interdependency of the human mind and body, you sometimes get benefits from a therapeutic action just because you believe you will. Physicians first observed this phenomenon while testing whether particular substances were biologically active. Part of a group of test subjects received a potential drug, and, for control, the other half received a pharmacologically inert substance called a *placebo* (often a sugar pill). None of the test subjects, however, knew exactly which substance they received. In any type of experiment, some subjects who were taking the placebo showed an improvement in symptoms. This response became known as the *placebo effect.*

The placebo effect is not phony or bad; it's just a fact of human psychology. Most people can, and often do, use it positively. Your admirable attachment to teddy bears is a case in point. What is a teddy bear? Objectively, it's just cloth pieced together and stuffed. Can a stuffed bear reach out and give you a hug? Can you fend off the monsters of the night? Yet as children (and beyond), virtually everyone has drawn immense comfort from their teddies during times of stress or anxiety. On a more complex level, similar things are happening when people search for treatments for what ails them.

Western medicine tests potential medicines and therapies by conducting scientific trials designed to control for the placebo effect. Until only recently, few techniques or substances in alternative medicine were put through this type of controlled scientific trial. Although that doesn't mean some substances cannot have benefit, you nevertheless always need to sort through the evidence as best you can and educate yourself to determine which substances and techniques in alternative medicine have proven benefits.

Drawing on Lifestyle Medicine and the Mind/Body Connection

If you look at various lists of alternative therapies from a variety of sources, you're likely to find the lifestyle practices that you probably think of as mainstream right at the top of the list — sound nutrition, appropriate physical activity and exercise, and stress reduction, for example. In fact, these once-alternative therapies have become mainstream medicine because a huge body of evidence proves that many daily habits and practices in these areas clearly lower your risks of heart disease and help you manage many heart conditions. At the same time, each of these proven lifestyle measures offers an *alternative* that often can render advanced cardiac techniques or medicines used in Western medicine unnecessary or can serve as a *complement* to such techniques.

Three areas of lifestyle medicine are so important that I've devoted a chapter to each: See Chapter 20 on nutrition and weight management, Chapter 21 on physical activity, and Chapter 22 on reducing stress.

In this section, I discuss additional mind/body techniques that you may find useful in helping reduce your risk of heart disease or managing your heart disease to achieve the quality of life you desire.

Tapping mind/body techniques

No other organ in the body, with the possible exception of the brain, is more affected by your emotional state than the heart. Profound mind/body connections impact everything from hypertension to cardiac rhythms. In addition to the techniques for stress reduction that I discuss in Chapter 22, here are several mind/body techniques that can be useful as part of a positive lifestyle.

- **Biofeedback:** Several forms of biofeedback may be useful in promoting relaxation and stress reduction. In particular, using a heart rate monitor to assist individuals with relaxation exercises — such as the 10-minute timeout described in Chapter 22 — and with promoting heart health and safety by monitoring aerobic physical activity using target heart rate zones. Such biofeedback is effective in enhancing a number of stress-reduction and exercise techniques.

- **Tai chi:** This ancient Chinese discipline combines movement, deep breathing, and meditation, is appropriate for all ages, and can be adapted to all fitness levels. As your physical conditioning progresses, you can progress in the difficulty or duration of the tai chi exercises. Studies show that tai chi may be particularly useful in helping older patients improve balance, strength, flexibility, and cardiovascular fitness. Recognizing its benefits, many medical health centers provide tai chi classes as part of their wellness programs.

- **Yoga:** Yoga, which originated in India, combines movement (including stretching and poses) with breathing exercises and meditation to achieve relaxation and better flexibility, muscle strength, and functional health. Among the many styles of yoga are gentle forms that are appropriate for people with heart disease and perhaps other physical limitations. One benefit of yoga is that you can then advance as your conditioning improves. Many medical health centers provide yoga classes as part of their wellness and rehabilitation programs.

Individuals with heart disease need to avoid beginning yoga with one of the newly popular forms that emphasize rigorous, aerobic workouts. Instead, start with a gentle, relaxation-oriented class tailored to beginners.

Is natural better?

In recent years, natural products have developed quite a stamp of approval. Now, I'm all for natural products. Eating fruits and vegetables is the most natural way of getting fiber and many antioxidants and vitamins, particularly vitamin C.

Some of the most important drugs were developed from plant sources. You may even have the source of digitalis, one of the first and most important medicines for heart rhythm problems, growing in your garden right now. The foxglove plants brightening your yard used to be ground up to produce a powder containing digitalis. Scientists later were able achieve even better results by purifying these same compounds in the laboratory. So the current medication known as *digoxin* leads straight back to foxglove and shares the same chemistry.

That leads to my last point:: Just because a product is natural doesn't mean that it's better than a similar product that has been synthesized. Natural is neutral. Simply describing a product as "natural" does not qualify it as beneficial or ineffective nor as safe or harmful. Natural products, by their nature, haven't been subjected to the same purification processes that other products (approved medicines included) have undergone. That doesn't mean all natural products should be avoided. On the contrary, it simply means that consumers need to be aware that natural does not necessarily mean better or safer. Likewise, synthesized does not necessarily mean a product is not natural or that it doesn't have natural origins. As always, do your homework and use your common sense.

Opening up to spirituality

Although it may be splitting hairs, I separate spirituality from mind/body techniques. Both, however, are aspects of your psychological makeup. The degree of importance spirituality has on your outlook on life and perhaps even on your cardiovascular health is amazing. Two cases in point:

- ✔ **The power of prayer:** One recent study revealed that more than 95 percent of the people undergoing coronary artery bypass grafting engaged in prayer the evening before. I think placing more emphasis on understanding and respecting the spirituality of patients in modern cardiovascular medicine is not only good for health-care givers as human beings but also enhances the outcomes of many of the procedures that they undertake.

- ✔ **The power of gardening:** Major studies show that people who garden regularly lower their risk of heart disease. Although gardeners may get a little exercise every day, it typically isn't enough to account for all the benefit. I think on some profound level, gardeners are getting a dose of spirituality as they tend other living things. Gardeners are optimists who plant seeds in spring, confident of the crops they'll produce in the summer and fall. Without a doubt, my patients who are gardeners seem to do better than the ones who don't have this connection with life and the earth.

Volunteering

My favorite song in the Disney movie *The Lion King* is "Circle of Life." This song reminds me that everyone is connected to each other in the circle of life. Recent studies show that people who work as volunteers and help others actually improve their own health. Isn't it wonderful to know that following your natural inclination to connect with other people and do good generates better health as a totally unintended side benefit?

Looking at How Natural Supplements May Help Combat Heart Disease

Ten years ago, I would've joined most physicians in saying that if you eat a balanced and healthy diet and meet all of the recommended daily allowances of vitamins and minerals, you probably don't need any supplements. However, within only the last five years, a number of studies have persuaded me that there are situations in which supplementation may be appropriate. At the same time, many issues still need to be explored, so I recommend that you consider supplementation on a case-by-case basis and that you explore the issues with your cardiologist before taking any supplements. In addition, find out as much as you can about any given supplement and its potential role in cardiovascular and total health and its potential for negative interaction with other medicines you may be taking.

The sections that follow discuss some of the more popular natural supplements currently available and whether enough evidence exists to recommend them as substances that can lower your risk of heart disease or play a role in helping you fight heart disease.

Phytosterols

Phytosterols, which are plant substances chemically related to cholesterol, help fight heart disease by binding onto cholesterol in the intestines and thus preventing it from being absorbed. More than 50 phytosterols have been identified in nature and enrich many different foods, including legumes (peas and kidney beans, in particular), wheat germ, oranges, bananas, Brussels sprouts, and cauliflower.

For optimal results, you need to consume phytosterol-rich foods with meals, because the act of mechanically binding to cholesterol is what gives them their cholesterol-lowering properties. Phytosterols are another good reason for eating at least five servings of fruits and vegetables daily. Phytosterol may even sound cool enough to convince your kids to try a Brussels sprout.

Red yeast rice (monascus purpureus)

Red yeast rice contains an active agent known as *monascus purpureus* that comes from the ancient Chinese herbal medicine chest and recently was subjected to rigorous trials by Western science. The results are impressive. In fact, they're so impressive that the U.S. Food and Drug Administration (FDA) classified monascus purpureus as a drug that is pharmacologically related to the class of cholesterol-lowering drugs called *statins*. Because the FDA considers it a powerful drug, red yeast rice may no longer be sold legally in the United States as a food supplement. The best advice is to avoid taking this supplement.

Garlic

Beloved in all the world's cuisines, garlic was touted for its medicinal benefits more than 5,000 years ago in Sanskrit records from ancient India. Hippocrates wrote about garlic's use, and so did the Chinese. More recently, garlic has been promoted as a way of lowering cholesterol and triglycerides. Be careful with this one, though, because the most recent studies haven't proven garlic's cholesterol-lowering capabilities. (But garlic's still great for tasty heart-healthy eating; I love garlic and use it regularly to make great-tasting, low-fat dishes.)

Garlic may, however, have other medicinal benefits. Some studies suggest that it may contain substances that inhibit blood clotting, which, of course, can be beneficial in terms of lowering the risk of heart attack and stroke. For now, the jury is out on garlic as a beneficial cardiovascular supplement and research continues. If you're among the many people who enjoy the taste of garlic, cooking with it certainly can't hurt and may help, but I wouldn't recommend taking any garlic supplements in pill or powdered form without first discussing it with your cardiologist or primary-care physician.

Niacin

Niacin is a B vitamin that long has been known as essential for preventing *pellagra,* a condition characterized by skin inflammation and gastrointestinal disturbances. More recent studies show that niacin also reduces total cholesterol levels while increasing HDL, the good cholesterol. Decreases in LDL (the bad cholesterol) of between 20 percent and 30 percent, combined with increases in protective HDL of 20 percent, frequently have been associated with niacin. In fact, niacin is one of the few substances that lowers LDL and, at the same time, raises HDL. Cardiologists now use it as a mainstay in therapy to lower cholesterol.

Folate

Folate is another B vitamin that is thought to lower *homocysteine,* a dangerous form of amino acid in the blood. High homocysteine levels have been associated with increased risk of heart disease. I believe that the evidence is strong enough to recommend that every adult man and woman consume 400 micrograms of folate every day. Although green leafy vegetables and citrus fruits contain high levels of folate, simply eating fruits and vegetables is rarely enough to bring your folate intake to the recommended level. The best advice is to take either a multivitamin with folate or consume a fully fortified cereal such as Total every day to get your daily dosage of folate.

Fiber

Dietary fiber occurs in two major forms: soluble and insoluble.

Soluble fiber combines with water and fluids in the intestine to form gels that can absorb other substances and trap them. The trapped substances include bile acids that contain large amounts of cholesterol. Thus, consuming soluble fiber is a particularly good way of lowering cholesterol, because as bile acids are excreted from the body, the liver uses up cholesterol to make more bile acids.

So much strong evidence supports this function of soluble fiber that the FDA allows certain foods that are rich in soluble fiber to claim that when they're used in conjunction with a low-fat diet, they may further lower your risk of heart disease. Oatmeal and whole-oat, ready-to-eat cereals are perhaps the most prominent among such foods that are eaten regularly.

Insoluble fiber may also provide health benefits that are not related to heart disease. For example, this type of fiber helps trap water in the stools, providing more bulk and helping food move through the digestive system more quickly. This effect may help lower the risk of colon cancer.

The American Heart Association and National Cancer Institute recommend consuming 25 grams of fiber daily. Most people consume only about 12 grams. Thus, I strongly recommend that you try to increase the amount of fiber in your diet. High-fiber foods such as bran, beans, oatmeal, and many cereals are excellent sources of fiber, and so are many fruits and vegetables. Some fiber supplements, such as Metamucil and Citrucel, also may help.

Common-sense checklist for evaluating alternative therapies

So how do you sort through all the claims, evidence, information, and sometimes heated rhetoric about particular alternative products or techniques? Asking these questions may help you find and evaluate the information you need to make wise decisions:

✔ When researching a specific therapy (particularly a controversial one), have you reviewed the arguments and evidence from all sides of the issue?

✔ What evidence supports the effectiveness of the therapy?

Have scientific trials been conducted or is the support based only on testimony and anecdote?

Is the support based on quantifiable data or opinion?

How old, how large, and how well-designed were any scientific trials? (Good science always pushes the envelope, reevaluates, seeks to acquire more data, and, when necessary, changes its mind. A few scientific trials from the 1920s or 1950s that are unsupported by more recent studies or that are even contradicted by later studies would not be the best evidence of the effectiveness of a given substance or technique.)

✔ How safe is the therapy?

Is there concrete evidence (not just a provider's or recipient's opinion) that the benefits outweigh the risks?

Does evidence suggest that the product does no harm when used as directed?

Under what conditions is service or treatment delivered?

✔ What credentials and expertise does the practitioner of an alternative therapy or developer of a product have? (A mail-order PhD from a diploma mill won't inspire confidence in the developer of the "SuperDooper Mighty-Mineral Supplement," will it?)

✔ What is the cost of the treatment or product?

✔ Have you discussed the therapy with your primary-care physician and cardiologist? If you're actually using the therapy, have you told your doctor? Your doctor needs a complete picture to give you the best health-care, including guarding against negative interactions with your other medicines or therapies. Many doctors are also good sources of information.

Soy protein

Some cultures have prized soy protein for its health benefits since ancient times. Modern science confirms that the type of protein found in soybeans has a complete set of *amino acids,* which are the building blocks for the body's protein. Soy protein also seems to lower cholesterol and is thought to carry antioxidants that may help prevent heart disease in ways other than simply by lowering cholesterol levels. If you enjoy the taste of soy, you can consume extra soy protein by drinking soybean milk, using soy-based meat substitutes, or sampling the many new soy products that recently entered the marketplace.

Fish oil

Why do certain cultures that consume large quantities of cold-water fish (the Eskimo culture, for instance) have low incidences of heart disease? The reason seems related to the oils that these fish contain. These oils are high in a substance called omega-3 fatty acids. A number of studies show that cholesterol levels can be lowered by as much as 10 percent when fish is substituted for red meat in the diet two to three times per week. What a good reason to enjoy fish. I strongly recommend it. You'll get an excellent source of high-level protein that may, in addition, contain these cholesterol-lowering substances. One word of caution, however: Evidence is inconclusive about the benefits of taking fish oil supplements rather than actually eating the fish.

Antioxidants

Antioxidants are thought to decrease the likelihood that LDL cholesterol will be oxidized. If this finding is borne out by continuing research, antioxidants may prove useful because the oxidized form of LDL cholesterol is what appears to do the most damage. Recommended antioxidants include vitamin C, vitamin E, and beta carotene. The doses that seem to be necessary to yield these potential cardiac benefits are vitamin C 250 to 500 mg a day and vitamin E 200 to 400 IU (International Units) per day.

But any definite conclusions about the benefits of antioxidants remain up in the air. Although early trials indicated that antioxidants lower your risk of heart disease, more recent trials haven't confirmed that finding. For people with certain heart conditions, beta carotene also appears to carry a risk. So what would I do? I usually tell patients who do not have contraindications (reasons they shouldn't use them) that I don't object to their taking antioxidants, but I also point out that a definitive answer about the role they may play in combating the risk of heart disease (or risk of any other disease) has not yet been found.

Part V
Living Well with Heart Disease

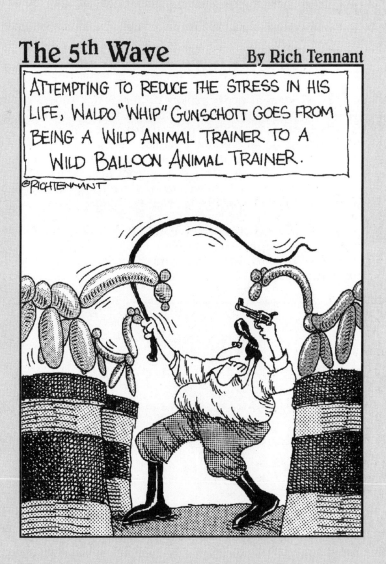

The 5th Wave   By Rich Tennant

ATTEMPTING TO REDUCE THE STRESS IN HIS LIFE, WALDO "WHIP" GUNSCHOTT GOES FROM BEING A WILD ANIMAL TRAINER TO A WILD BALLOON ANIMAL TRAINER.

@RICHTENNANT

In this part . . .

Here's your chance to explore the reality that you can live well with heart disease by using a number of strategies to prevent, control, and sometimes reverse it. First, I detail the ways in which cardiac rehabilitation can help you return to full, productive living after a heart attack or heart surgery. Then, I show you evidence that combining powerful lifestyle practices with modern medical therapies may enable you to halt or even reverse the progress of coronary heart disease. Finally, I share the basic principles, strategies, and tips that you need to work with your physician to adopt nutritional practices, a physical activity plan, and stress reduction strategies that will help you fight heart disease.

Chapter 18

Rehabilitating Your Heart

• •

In This Chapter

▶ Discovering cardiac rehabilitation

▶ Defining the goals and benefits of cardiac rehabilitation

▶ Using exercise and physical activity in cardiac rehabilitation

▶ Identifying strategies for long-term success

• •

*W*ould it surprise you to know that only 25 percent of the people who can benefit from cardiac rehabilitation programs actually participate in them? What an enormous and tragic waste that 75 percent of the people who are eligible miss out on the following benefits of cardiac rehabilitation programs:

✔ Improved exercise tolerance and ability to carry out activities of daily living.

✔ Reduced symptoms such as angina and shortness of breath.

✔ Improved cholesterol and blood lipid levels.

✔ Reduced cigarette smoking.

✔ Improved sense of well-being.

✔ Reduced stress.

✔ Reduced mortality. Heart attack victims who participate in rehabilitation programs experience a 25 percent reduction in mortality during the first three years after their heart attacks when compared with those who don't participate.

Understanding Cardiac Rehabilitation

Cardiac rehabilitation is a long-term program with several therapeutic components designed to help individuals get better after a variety of heart problems, angioplasty, or cardiac surgery. It is an important tool in what physicians call *secondary prevention* of heart disease, which is prevention of another heart event after you've had one.

Specific plans and components of a cardiac rehabilitation program usually are tailored to the specific conditions and needs of each patient; however, all cardiac rehabilitation programs need to include these four areas, which I explain in detail later in the chapter:

- Education about your cardiac condition and treatment
- Exercise training and physical activity prescriptions
- Lifestyle modifications to reduce risk factors for heart disease
- Counseling and support

Although individual prescriptions for cardiac rehabilitation vary according to each individual patient's condition, the goals and benefits always remain the same:

- Educating you about how to control your cardiac condition
- Reducing the heart's disability and improving its ability to function in a way that supports your ability to carry out life's daily activities effectively and independently
- Decreasing the likelihood that you'll experience further problems from your cardiac condition and perhaps even decreasing the need for heart medicines
- Identifying and providing ways to modify risk factors that may result in continued problems from various forms of heart disease
- Increasing the likelihood that an individual will return to work and a full, happy, and long life following a cardiac event

Discovering just who needs cardiac rehabilitation

Modern cardiac rehabilitation programs are an important component of an overall care plan for many patients with heart disease and, more specifically, in these seven circumstances:

- When diagnosed with coronary artery disease (CAD)/angina
- Following a heart attack
- Following coronary artery bypass surgery
- Following coronary angioplasty
- Following heart surgery on the valves
- Before and following heart transplantation
- When experiencing heart failure

As you can see from this list, the vast majority of people with heart disease can benefit from cardiac rehabilitation.

Exploring Varied Cardiac Rehabilitation Components

Formal, medically supervised cardiac rehabilitation programs usually take place either in the hospital or in the community. These programs offer a great advantage: Everything you need to improve your cardiac health can be found in one place, and knowledgeable medical staff members are on hand at all times to provide you with educational support, ensure your safety, and keep you motivated.

If you've been hospitalized for a heart attack, cardiac surgery, or other problem, your rehabilitation program starts while you're in the hospital. After you're discharged, you typically continue your program on an outpatient basis by participating in either a hospital- or community-sponsored cardiac rehabilitation program.

Unfortunately, some people are unable to participate in formal cardiac rehabilitation programs, because they live so far away from the centers where programs are provided. With advancing communications technology, many hospitals and cardiologists are beginning to offer new home-based rehabilitation programs that use telephone-based supervision and communication with participants. Such home-based programs are intended only for people with stable cardiac conditions who are at low or moderate risk of developing further problems.

Ideally, you will continue to work on your *rehab* for the rest of your life, because the information, strategies, and techniques you use during rehabilitation give you excellent tools for living long and well overall and not just for retooling the old ticker. That said, formal cardiac rehabilitation programs usually have three phases:

1. **Rehabilitation during hospitalization**

2. **Formal supervised rehabilitation program during recovery**

3. **Maintenance program**

Starting rehabilitation while you're in the hospital

If you're hospitalized for a cardiac problem or surgery, your rehabilitation begins during your stay in the hospital.

Members of the rehabilitation team begin counseling you on your cardiac condition and how to manage it. Topics may include nutrition, weight reduction (if necessary), stress reduction, stopping smoking, and other lifestyle modifications. You also begin supervised physical therapy and physical activity.

When doctors deem you ready to go home, your medical team makes sure that you receive instructions for what you need to do at home to continue your progress. Your doctor usually recommends when you should begin a medically supervised cardiac rehabilitation program. The timing depends on your particular situation and condition, but, in general, you'll be ready to start in one to three weeks.

In the meantime, you're not supposed to be idle at home. You need to continue with the physical activities, exercises, and diet your physician recommends for your recovery. In some instances, your physician may prescribe home visits from a social worker or physical therapist to help you out.

Continuing rehabilitation during recovery

After your initial recovery, you begin participating in a medically supervised cardiac rehabilitation program. Typical cardiac rehabilitation programs feature group and individual exercises, along with a variety of educational programs that help lower your risk factors for heart disease.

Your physical activity usually includes aerobic exercise on a treadmill, a stationary cycle, or a walking track. However, equipment and activities also are available for people with walking difficulties to build their aerobic capacity. Enhancing mobility is, after all, a goal. The physical activity starts slowly — to ensure safety — but gradually builds to a more intensive program.

During your exercise program, your heart rate, blood pressure, and, at least in the early stages, electrical impulses and rhythm of your heart as indicated by an electrocardiogram ECG are monitored by a nurse or other health-care professional to make sure you're not having any problems.

Strength training, in some instances, may be included in your program. Proper instruction and supervision are crucial, and strength training is not advised for all cardiac conditions.

Most rehabilitation programs include classes in nutrition, risk-factor reduction, weight management (if necessary), smoking cessation, and stress management education. Access to counseling, educational materials, and support groups also is likely to be available for:

✔ Job and vocational guidance to help you with returning to work

✔ Physical capabilities and limitations, including (but not limited to) when you can start having sexual relations, how much exertion you can take in daily life, and so on

✔ Psychological and emotional matters

Although your physician recommends the length of time you should participate in a cardiac rehabilitation program, 6 to 12 weeks usually is the minimum. A number of studies, however, indicate that heart rehab patients who participate for periods of from three to six months to a year experience even greater improvements.

Maintaining your program to keep gaining benefits

Continuing your physical activity program and sustaining and strengthening your new nutritional and lifestyle practices are important for maintaining and increasing the gains you achieve during your formal rehab program. In fact, "keeping on keeping on" is the key to unlocking the lasting benefits of cardiac rehabilitation.

Educating Yourself about Your Heart Condition

Being diagnosed with heart disease, experiencing a heart attack, or undergoing heart surgery is scary. In fact, it's so scary that you may try to avoid thinking about your condition — you just want to get over it and get back to your old life. Or it's so scary that thinking positively about the future is difficult. Fear, denial, anger, and all the other emotional reactions to heart disease or a cardiac event are normal. The first and foremost tool for dealing with them is knowledge. That's why helping you educate yourself about your particular condition is an important component of rehabilitation programs.

Finding out as much as you can about your condition, how to manage it, how to reduce any resulting limitations, and how to enhance abilities can unlock the door to a new freedom and a new discovery of what having a good life truly means. If you've had a heart event, *Heart Disease For Dummies* (in conjunction with the rehabilitation prescribed by your doctor) can help you become a knowledgeable, educated patient who is empowered to become an equal partner in his or her recovery and rehabilitation.

Exercising and Physical Activity as Part of Rehabilitation

Slowly progressive exercise training and physical activity programs and prescriptions represent the cornerstone of all modern cardiac rehabilitation programs. The benefits of such activity for people with heart disease are numerous, including:

- ✔ Increasing the efficiency and performance of the heart muscle itself.

- ✔ Increasing the efficiency of the exercising muscles, thereby reducing the workload that the heart must perform.

- ✔ Reducing the likelihood of further cardiac problems. This benefit is particularly true when such exercise programs are combined with risk-factor reduction and psychological support.

- ✔ Increasing your exercise capacity, which in turn can significantly improve your quality of life and result in a variety of other psychological benefits.

- ✔ Helping you feel that you're playing an active role in your recovery from heart disease.

Remember that as functional capacity increases after an acute heart problem, the likelihood of your returning to work and favorite activities increases.

Progressive exercise programs may also combat other risk factors for heart disease. For example, regular physical activity can significantly increase high-density lipoprotein (HDL — the good cholesterol), which is associated with decreased cardiac problems. In addition, regular physical activity can help with weight loss and may lower low-density lipoprotein (LDL — the bad kind of cholesterol), thereby further lowering the risk of future cardiac problems. (For more about cholesterol, check out Chapter 14.)

Getting started on an exercise program for rehab

In most instances, your doctor wants you to undergo some form of exercise tolerance test as part of the early process of cardiac rehabilitation. During that test, your doctor looks for evidence of inadequate blood flow to the heart, abnormal heart rhythms, or inadequate pumping action by the heart during exercise. Armed with this information, the doctor and other health-care workers can develop an individualized exercise program that enables you to achieve maximum benefits from exercise, while ensuring maximum safety.

After you suffer a cardiac event, exercise factors such as duration, intensity, and frequency of exercise are monitored carefully to ensure your safety as you begin exercising. Monitoring these factors ensures that your exercise program follows a slow progression toward helping to maximize your functional capacity and encouraging you to adopt a safe program that can be carried on for the rest of your life.

Modifying rehabilitative exercise training for specific conditions

Although basic principles of exercise training apply to all cardiac rehabilitation, some people with specific conditions require various modifications to the basic exercise-training program.

Patients with heart failure

Exercise programs in cardiac rehabilitation can be extremely helpful for people experiencing heart failure. Some studies show that people suffering from heart failure can improve their exercise capacity between 25 percent and 30 percent through controlled exercise programs. With those improvements typically come other improvements in the form of a better quality of life and decreased symptoms. The exercise prescription, however, needs to be modified in patients with heart failure because of their limited endurance. Lower target heart rates and intermittent rest periods enable them to slowly increase their endurance. Heart rates during exercise sessions typically are set at 10 beats per minute below the level at which any evidence of shortness of breath occurs. For a complete discussion about heart failure, turn to Chapter 7.

The elderly

People older than 65 who have cardiac problems and participate in cardiac rehabilitation can achieve significant improvements in their capacity to conduct activities of daily living. In one study, functional capacity increased by 50 percent. Although exercise programs may need to be modified to accommodate limited endurance, elderly individuals stand to gain the most from cardiac rehabilitation. Yet this group nevertheless is among the most underserved.

Patients with heart rhythm problems

Patients who have been hospitalized with heart rhythm problems may benefit from cardiac rehabilitation programs. Because these people may be at particularly high risk for problems during cardiac rehabilitation, however, they require

✔ Supervision by doctors who are knowledgeable about their specific rhythm problems

✔ Appropriate medications to suppress rhythm disturbances

✔ Longer periods of continuous monitoring (using electrocardiograms) than individuals who haven't had cardiac rhythm problems

Women

Although women experience the same benefits of exercise training as men during cardiac rehabilitation, women are significantly less likely to be referred for cardiac rehabilitation. This shortfall is particularly unfortunate because more than half of all deaths from coronary artery disease (CAD) now occur in women. Women are also more likely than men to experience other problems, including death, following a heart attack. Thus, cardiac rehabilitation is particularly important for women. So, ladies, insist on it or find out why it isn't recommended.

Cardiac transplantation patients

Research shows that cardiac rehabilitation is highly effective for cardiac transplantation patients, helping increase their endurance and capacity to perform activities of daily living. A number of changes in the cardiovascular system occur following cardiac transplantation. These changes often require modifications to typical cardiac rehabilitation programs. For example, the response of a transplanted heart to exercise is different in terms of heart rate than in a nontransplanted heart. During the transplantation process, all the nerves that serve the normal heart are severed. The result is a difference in how the reattached nerves send signals to the heart. Therefore, heart transplant patients need to be involved in programs with an experienced rehabilitation team whose members are skilled in their particular exercise prescription.

Coronary artery bypass surgery or heart attack patients

Astonishingly, only an estimated 15 percent of the patients who can benefit from cardiac rehabilitation following heart attack or coronary artery bypass surgery ever actually are involved in formal cardiac rehabilitation programs. This low rate of participation probably is a result of a combination of factors, including:

✔ Inadequate referrals by physicians

✔ Poor patient motivation

✔ Financial considerations

✔ Logistical issues, such as being too far away (or otherwise inconvenient) from major cardiac rehabilitation centers or inconvenience

If you or a loved one is in this situation, making that extra effort to get involved in a cardiac rehabilitation program is important so you can derive the multiple benefits.

Developing Strategies for Long-Term Success

How successful any rehabilitation program is in lowering your risk of future cardiac events relates directly to how conscientiously you follow the program.

Cardiac rehabilitation has many benefits and minimal risks. Comprehensive cardiac rehabilitation programs help you or a loved one fight back against heart disease. The biggest risk is not participating at all. Ask your doctor whether cardiac rehabilitation is appropriate for you, and when it is, take advantage of this potentially lifesaving part of modern cardiac care.

Assessing in your own mind and heart, discussing all the potential benefits of cardiac rehabilitation with your family and physician, and developing a strategy for sticking with it in the long run (or long walk!) are important steps to take. The formal rehabilitation program may end, but your work is never done.

Modifying your lifestyle to reduce the risks of additional heart problems

Risk-factor reduction is particularly important for patients who have heart disease and/or who have undergone cardiac surgery. Cardiac rehabilitation programs need to place particular emphasis on blood pressure control, proper nutritional counseling, weight reduction (if the patient is overweight), and smoking cessation.

✔ **Blood pressure control:** Managing your blood pressure by keeping it within normal levels can reduce your risk of further problems and complications from your heart disease. Adhering to a multifaceted approach that includes education, diet modifications, a program of physical activity, stress reduction, and prescribed medications is important. (For more about hypertension, see Chapter 13.)

✔ **Nutritional counseling:** Strong evidence exists that lowering blood cholesterol and improving lipoprotein profiles are extremely beneficial for people with CAD. The principles behind the Eating Plan for Healthy Americans and TLC Diet (see Chapters 14 and 20) form the foundation for nutritional counseling in cardiac rehabilitation programs. Seeking such nutritional instruction from a registered dietitian is important. Remember, sodium-restricted diets are appropriate for patients with high blood pressure or heart failure.

✔ **Weight control:** Studies show that losing weight and maintaining weight at appropriate levels can help people with heart disease control high blood pressure, improve and even normalize their cholesterol levels, and control the risk of diabetes. Weight loss also contributes to improving your ability to comfortably carry out daily activities (see Chapter 20).

✔ **Smoking cessation:** Without a doubt, patients with CAD who continue to smoke have a higher likelihood of suffering further complications or even death. The converse also is also true. Patients who stop smoking after a heart attack reduce their risk of further cardiac events. (See also Chapter 23.)

Getting some counseling and support

The majority of patients who've suffered an acute problem from heart disease experience one or more psychological problems. Common conditions include

✔ **Moderate to severe depression:** Following a heart attack, up to 20 percent of patients experience this kind of depression. Likewise, up to 10 percent of them face significant anxiety disorders that require therapy.

✔ **A reduction in sexual activity:** In fact, almost 25 percent of heart attack patients never resume sexual activity and more than 50 percent decrease their sexual activity following a heart attack.

✔ **Family and marital problems and social isolation:** These problems are common sequels to heart disease.

People with severe heart disease commonly go through a cycle of fear that often leads to anger and ultimately to depression. Some of the more common feelings are

✔ Fear that you're dying

✔ Fear that chest pains will recur

✔ Fear that you'll never return to work

✔ Fear that you'll never have sex again

✔ Anger that a heart problem happened to you

✔ Anger at yourself for not changing conditions that may or may not have been under your control that ultimately resulted in the heart problem

✔ Anger with family and friends

✔ Depression at the thought that your "life is over" (or will never be the same again)

✔ Depression at the idea that others may think you're weak or damaged goods

Psychological counseling can help in all of these situations, particularly during the early phases of recovery, and it therefore needs to be a part of all cardiac rehabilitation programs. Participating in a support group with other people who've experienced problems or have conditions similar to yours can be beneficial. You can find support groups online. Ask your cardiologist or a member of the staff at your rehabilitation center whether they know of groups in your area.

Support from counselors also can help you establish positive interactive links with your family and friends. A number of rehab programs offer support groups and educational classes for family members that can enhance the recovery of your entire family. Yes, heart problems affect more than the victim who suffers from them.

Safely returning to work

One benefit of cardiac rehabilitation is that trained professionals can help guide anyone who has suffered from a heart problem in making important decisions, such as determining whether and when to return to work, choosing whether to change the type of work you do, and assessing the risks of having further problems if you return to work.

Your physician often is guided by the results of objective tests, such as the treadmill exercise test. The results of such tests, in conjunction with the physical demands of your job, help guide you and your medical team in deciding whether and when you return to work. The exact nature of your work, whether it involves strenuous labor, and particularly whether it involves work with your arms and chest, are important issues to discuss with your physician. Be sure that you talk to your doctor about the nature and levels of stress that are typical of your work.

The good news: Most people can return to work following most acute heart problems, and cardiac rehab helps that happen sooner.

Partnering with your physician

If you think you or a loved one is eligible for and can benefit from cardiac rehabilitation, *talk to your doctor.* If your doctor isn't willing to consider cardiac rehabilitation for you and you think you're eligible, obtaining a second opinion may be worthwhile.

Some questions to ask your doctor include

✔ Am I eligible for cardiac rehabilitation?

✔ Is cardiac rehabilitation covered by my health insurance?

✔ Where is the nearest cardiac rehabilitation program?

✔ How often do I need to go to cardiac rehabilitation sessions?

✔ How long should I participate in a cardiac rehabilitation program?

✔ What benefits can I expect from a cardiac rehabilitation program?

Finding More Information

If you think that you or a loved one may be eligible for cardiac rehabilitation, talk to your physician, nurse, or health-care professional. You can also obtain information from your local chapter of the American Heart Association (AHA) by calling 800-242-8721, and you can read more about cardiac rehabilitation on the AHA Web site at www.americanheart.org.

Chapter 19

Reversing Heart Disease: Hope or Hype?

In This Chapter

▶ Understanding why regress means progress

▶ Identifying the route to reversing heart disease

▶ Defining a practical approach for turning CAD around

When Thomas Wolfe's famous novel *You Can't Go Home Again* came out in 1940, most people thought his title had hit on one true thing. For many years, cardiologists believed that same truth applied to coronary artery disease: Once you had this progressive, relentless condition, you might be able to slow down the process, but you couldn't actually reverse it — you couldn't go home again.

But in medicine, as in life, the quest to go home again continues. Cardiologists now know that *yes*, you can do a number of things that can halt the progression of coronary artery disease (CAD) in its tracks — at least for most people. If you have CAD and want to make this happen, however, you're going to have to stop cold and make major changes in how you eat, exercise, work, and generally live your life. You usually have to take lipid-lowering (cholesterol and other fat) medicines, too. But as long as you're willing to do your part and adopt these strict measures, you can look forward to more hope than hype in the promise that you can reverse coronary artery disease (CAD). In fact, an estimated 50 percent to 60 percent of those who go this route actually experience some reversal of their CAD.

Before going any further, I want to emphasize two points. If you're thinking that, given the good news in this chapter, you can live a life of sin (sloth and gluttony of the seven deadlies come to mind) and then later repent and turn the negative health effects around, forget about it! Preventing heart disease still is always be better than to trying to reverse it.

Likewise, this chapter is not a do-it-yourself manual. You need to work with your cardiologist. Having CAD means that you have a dangerous condition. Even in the best outcomes, only 50 percent to 60 percent of individuals who stringently follow the regimens outlined in this chapter actually experience some reversal of their heart disease. Some individuals experience a halt in the progression of their CAD (also a very good thing!), while 20 percent to 30 percent continue to experience a progression of CAD, despite their best efforts. For all these reasons, it is critically important for you not to try to go it alone.

Turning Back Time

Can coronary artery disease regress? The simple answer to this question is *yes*. A number of studies show that under the right circumstances, 50 percent to 60 percent of narrowing of coronary arteries can actually be reversed, at least to some degree.

Differing approaches have been used in various studies, but the cumulative results to date support one central therapeutic strategy. These findings indicate that by diminishing the amount of lipid (cholesterol and fats) within the plaque (the fatty deposits that narrow your coronary arteries), you can decrease the likelihood that the plaque will rupture and thus set in process the catastrophic sequence of events that leads to unstable angina or heart attack. (See Chapter 4 to review how plaque formation takes place.)

Looking at evidence of CAD regression

Since 1990, more than 20 major scientific studies have shown that regression of coronary artery disease can occur. These studies can be grouped into four therapeutic approaches.

- **Diet or diet plus other interventions:** Five major studies were conducted during the last 20 years using either diet alone, diet in combination with other lifestyle factors, or, in several instances, low-fat diet in combination with medicines. The results of these studies are quite consistent:

  - In cases where cholesterol is lowered more than 25 percent, and LDL cholesterol (the bad guys) in particular is lowered more than 30 percent, at least some degree of regression of CAD has occurred in approximately half of the patients participating in the study.

  - When total cholesterol is lowered by between 10 percent and 20 percent, regression of coronary artery disease occurs in about one-third of patients.

- **Intervention with a single drug to lower lipids:** In the studies where drug therapy was used to lower lipids as a mechanism to promote regression of coronary artery disease, the results again are consistent:

If total cholesterol is lowered more than 20 percent, and LDL cholesterol is lowered approximately 30 percent, anywhere from 30 percent to 50 percent of participating patients experience regression of the CAD or at least a halt of progression.

✔ **Combinations of drugs to lower lipids:** Four studies used a combination of drug interventions to lower cholesterol. Once again, the results are quite promising. Approximately one-half of the participating patients experienced either regression or a halt in progression of CAD, provided that they significantly lowered their total cholesterol and LDL cholesterol. Likewise, the levels of HDL cholesterol (the good guys) in some patients actually increased.

✔ **Other interventions to lower lipids:** One study used surgery to lower cholesterol in an attempt to cause regression of coronary artery disease. In this study, part of the small bowel was bypassed to decrease the absorption of fats. In this situation, 50 percent to 60 percent of patients who had the surgery experienced either regression of CAD or a halt in its progression.

Offering a promising outlook and a caution

Although cumulative evidence from these studies is very hopeful, and ongoing research should help doctors discover more about therapies that may help their patients halt and regress CAD, the state of the art is, well, far from being state of the art. No matter how many individuals improve as a result of these trials, you need to remember that as many as 20 percent to 30 percent of them actually experience a progression of their CAD in spite of significant lowering of their lipid levels.

Considering How Coronary Artery Disease Regresses

The studies discussed in the previous section also provide evidence that these therapies work to reverse CAD by boosting and reinforcing the body's natural healing process.

In the same way that an injury to the vessel wall stimulates the formation of plaque that narrows the arteries, it also stimulates a number of natural processes that slowly attempt to heal the injury. Dramatic changes, such as a swift and significant reduction in LDL, appear to speed up these healing processes, thereby promoting regression of CAD.

Attacking the most dangerous plaque: The culprit lesions

The process of regressing CAD is particularly dramatic in attacking what cardiologists call culprit lesions. *Culprit lesions* are the types of plaques that usually commit the crime; they crack and thereby cause acute heart problems. Although culprit lesions account for only about 10 percent to 20 percent of all plaques, and usually present only mild or moderate narrowing of coronary arteries, they nevertheless appear to be responsible for between 80 percent and 90 percent of the episodes of unstable angina and heart attack. They're also characterized as having a great deal of lipids in their cores, which may be the central reason why they appear to be the kinds of plaque that stabilize when you dramatically lower cholesterol and other lipids.

Proving that regression has occurred

In the studies of the regression of coronary artery disease, researchers of course had to find ways to positively confirm whether the narrowing of coronary arteries had been reversed. That meant participants in earlier studies were required to undergo repeated heart catheterizations to take actual pictures of their coronary arteries — costly procedures that weren't much fun for the participants. The more recent studies used noninvasive techniques, such as PET scanning (see Chapter 11), which, although still costly (probably more costly than catheterizations), are less time-consuming and not as unpleasant for participants. These factors also point to similar reasons why only dozens and not hundreds of these important studies are conducted. Furthermore, a decrease in the number of acute heart events occurring after research participants received treatment also is considered indicative of probable stabilization or regression of CAD.

As a practical matter, if you're working with your doctor to reverse your own CAD, in all likelihood, you won't be required to go through these advanced tests. Instead, if you and your doctor are taking the steps that I recommend in the following section to dramatically lower your cholesterol in general and your LDL cholesterol in particular, you can assume with a reasonable degree of certainty that you're doing everything within your power to reverse your CAD.

Getting Practical about Reversing Coronary Artery Disease

So can you put all this cutting-edge research to work for you? I want to emphasize that this approach is no magic bullet, but yes, you can set in motion the processes that can reverse CAD — at least to a degree. If you conscientiously practice the following four steps while working with your physician as an ally, you may achieve real progress against this foe.

1. **Lower your lipids.**

   Lowering total cholesterol, and LDL cholesterol in particular, appears to be essential in reversing the process of atherosclerosis or clogging of the coronary arteries. Research is ongoing to settle the debate about what matters most in promoting regression — reaching an absolute level of LDL cholesterol below which regression occurs or achieving a certain percentage change of cholesterol and LDL cholesterol. Based on the best current evidence, I recommend that you try to lower your total cholesterol by about 20 percent and your LDL cholesterol by at least 30 percent to maximize your chances of starting the regression of CAD. I also believe that maintaining a total-cholesterol level below 170 and an LDL-cholesterol level below 100 is highly desirable.

   The two main ways to do this are

   - **By diet alone:** Several studies cited in this chapter use strict, low-fat, vegetarian diets. The diet advocated in the Lifestyle Heart Trial, for example, is an extremely low-fat diet with less than 10 percent of calories from fat, and significant reduction in saturated fat. Individuals who were able to stick with this very restricted diet lowered their total cholesterol by 24 percent and their LDL cholesterol by 37 percent. *Drawback:* This type of restricted diet is very difficult for most patients to follow.

   - **By diet and medication:** As a practical matter, most of the studies support combining a diet that derives less than 30 percent of its calories from fat and less than 10 percent of its calories from saturated fat (see the description of the AHA Eating Plan for Healthy Americans in Chapter 14) with one or more of the powerful lipid-lowering agents. Such an approach can lower lipid levels to the point where CAD regression begins. And most people may find it easier to stick with this approach than with the very low-fat diet alone. Of course, you need to work with your physician on this, and a registered dietitian who is skilled in administering low-fat diets should also be brought into the picture.

2. **Exercise regularly.**

   I am a strong advocate of regular exercise. Moderate exercise in conjunction with lowering other risk factors is known to lower your risk of secondary events from CAD; moreover, it needs to be part of any program designed to promote regression of CAD.

3. **Reduce stress.**

   The Lifestyle Heart Program, developed and popularized by Dr. Dean Ornish, emphasizes stress reduction as part of its overall model for regression of CAD. I'm a long-time advocate of mind/body interaction and think that stress reduction techniques such as visualization and meditation can play a significant role in the CAD regression. Many cardiologists, however, remain unconvinced of the value of these mind/body techniques for reversing heart disease.

4. **Work to reduce all your risk factors for CAD.**

The results of numerous studies reported in cardiac rehabilitation literature (see Chapter 18) show that a comprehensive approach to lowering risk factors for coronary artery disease results in significant decrease of the likelihood of recurrent complications. Controlling blood pressure, stopping cigarette smoking, and losing weight (if you're overweight) certainly are important ways to promote regression of CAD.

If you're one of the millions of Americans who suffer from CAD, your potential for reversing your illness represents the hope that you "can go home again," or at least turn around on the path and head toward home. But you must truly commit to the process. By that, I mean you have to be what one dignitary in a delightful slip of the tongue called *unswavering* (unswerving and unwavering). Then your body, in its infinite capacity for healing itself, can help you along the path toward regression.

Chapter 20

Choosing Heart-Healthy Nutrition and Managing Your Weight

As far as your heart goes, you are what you eat. Sound nutrition is critically important in maintaining and fostering heart health. Many people get hung up on one aspect of heart-healthy nutrition, such as lowering cholesterol. Although lowering cholesterol certainly is important (as discussed in Chapter 14), people often forget many other vital aspects of heart-healthy nutrition.

Warming Up to Nutrition — It Isn't a Four-Letter Word

The word *nutrition* grows out of an ancient Latin word meaning "to nourish" or "to suckle." How splendidly the root meaning of this word illustrates what eating well and eating right is all about, because mother's milk is a perfect blend of just the right amount of the nutrients that babies need for a good start. Likewise, good nutrition for all your and everyone else's lives means good eating from the balanced variety of foods needed to support life and health.

In spite of all the food and diet hype that you hear, the guidelines for healthy eating and weight management shared in this chapter are simple and can withstand the tests of experience and science. Adopting them as the foundation of your enjoyment of food points you toward a healthy heart and optimal health. So don't let the word *nutrition* scare you; just think good eating for good health.

Understanding you are what you eat: The bad news

Make no mistake, what you eat affects your health. The Surgeon General's Report on Nutrition and Health reminds everyone that eight of the ten leading causes of death in the United States have a nutrition or alcohol component. And heading the list as the number-one killer is cardiovascular disease — that's heart disease in simpler terms. In fact, overconsumption of dietary fat and calories and the inevitable results of added body fat are two major factors contributing to the continuing epidemic of heart disease in the U.S.

Understanding you are what you eat: The good news

Whatever trouble people eat themselves into, they generally can eat themselves out of! Even though poor food choices, such as eating too much dietary fat, contribute to significant health problems, including heart disease, adopting some simple, common-sense approaches to modifying your food choices for the better can lower your risk of heart disease and help you manage almost all heart conditions. These same smart choices also can help you control weight problems and improve health, happiness, and quality of life. These choices won't, however, bring back a good five-cent cup of coffee or improve the return on your IRA. You can't have everything.

Choosing Healthy Pleasures: Guidelines for Eating Right While Eating Well

Here's the first rule of heart-healthy eating: You can eat well in ways that improve your cardiac health without being a food cop.

Many people, however, suffer from the misconception that healthy cooking takes all the pleasure out of eating by making food taste bland and unappetizing. No way! In fact, many of the top chefs in America now are working with recipes that not only are healthy, low-fat variations but also are a pleasure to consume. Many home chefs are pretty expert, too — so why not you? Supporting you in this effort, I share ten heart-healthy recipes in the Appendix. They've been developed by some of America's top chefs. You can find a hundred more in *The Healthy Heart Cookbook For Dummies* (Wiley).

A number of major health and nutrition organizations in the U.S., including the American Heart Association (AHA) and the American Dietetic Association (ADA), have developed some basic principles for healthy nutrition. And they continue to refine these principles as new research adds to the literally thousands of scientific studies upon which they're based. The sections that follow are the essential nutritional goals to remember presented in simple, commonsensical statements.

Choose a variety of fruits and vegetables daily — at least five servings

Fruits and vegetables are important for what they do and do not contain. Fruits and vegetables are loaded with fiber, antioxidants, and other phytochemicals that lower the risks of heart disease and cancer. In addition, because they are low in sodium and most have no fat, fruits and vegetables don't increase blood cholesterol. Studies also show that people with high blood pressure who consume a diet containing high levels of fruits and vegetables and low-fat dairy products significantly reduced their blood pressure. Last, but hardly least, fruits and vegetables are a major source of the complex carbohydrates that are the body's primary source of fuel. For these reasons, every major, responsible nutritional organization recommends that people consume a minimum of five servings of fruits and vegetables per day. Shockingly, however, only 10 percent of the American public consumes this level of fruits and vegetables.

Choose a variety of whole-grain foods daily

Whole-grain products, such as cereals, breads, rice, and even pasta, form the mainstay of heart-healthy eating along with fruits and vegetables, because they are very high in fiber and in complex carbohydrates. Not consuming enough fiber clearly is associated with increased risk of heart disease. Everyone should be consuming approximately 25 grams of fiber from natural dietary sources every day, and yet the sad truth is that most folks eat only about half of this amount.

A tremendous amount of misinformation has reflected poorly on carbohydrates in the diet during the last few years. Many so-called experts have blamed carbohydrate consumption for the increased incidence of obesity in the U.S. Nothing could be further from the truth. *Overconsumption of calories,* coupled with *inadequate physical activity,* has led to the explosion of obesity in the U.S. Unfortunately, many of those extra calories have come from sugars or refined simple carbohydrates, which essentially are *empty calories,* or calories that don't provide the nutritional punch of whole-grain products. So think *whole-grain!*

Choose healthy fats in moderation and limit your intake of problem fats

Eating too much fat, particularly saturated fat (including transfat), contributes to two significant health problems: elevated cholesterol and obesity, which furthermore have clear links to increased risk of heart disease. A high-fat diet also is linked to diabetes and colon cancer. Moreover, eating lots of fat, which has nine calories per gram, compared with only four calories per gram for carbohydrates and protein, contributes to the overconsumption of calories by most Americans.

For these reasons, you need to set a goal of limiting the total amount of fat in your diet to less than 30 percent of total calories and, in particular, lowering the amount of saturated fat in your diet to less than 10 percent of total calories. Saturated fat needs to be restricted, because it contributes directly to elevating blood cholesterol and developing atherosclerosis, which often is called *hardening of the arteries* (see Chapter 4).

The three basic types of fat are

- ✔ **Saturated fat,** which typically comes from animal sources, although some fats from plants, such as cocoa butter, palm oil, and coconut oil also are saturated. Saturated fats typically are solid at room temperature. *Transfat*, which is hydrogenated or partially hydrogenated vegetable oil, also is saturated fat.

- ✔ **Monounsaturated fat,** which comes from vegetable sources, such as olive, canola, and peanut oils, and typically is liquid at room temperature. Substantial evidence suggests that monounsaturated fats, particularly the ways they are consumed in a Mediterranean diet that features olive oil, can significantly lower your risk of heart disease by raising HDL cholesterol without raising total cholesterol. See the nearby sidebar on Mediterranean diets.

- ✔ **Polyunsaturated fat,** which also comes primarily from vegetable sources and typically is liquid at room temperature. Corn oil and most other salad oils are examples of polyunsaturated oils. Unsaturated fats, however, can be turned into solid forms, and thus into a form of saturated fat known as transfat, through the process of *hydrogenation*. As a result of this process, many vegetable shortenings and stick margarines are high in saturated fat, even though the manufacturing process may have started with a polyunsaturated and/or monounsaturated oil.

Table 20-1 outlines the common food sources for each type of fat.

Table 20-1	Common Sources of Fats by Type	
Saturated Fats	*Monounsaturated Fats*	*Polyunsaturated Fats*
Animal Sources	**Animal Sources**	**Animal Sources (of omega-3 fatty acids)**
Cheese	Chicken	Fish
Butter	Fish	
Milk		**Plant Sources**
Meat (Beef, pork, chicken, lamb, and so on)	**Plant Sources**	Walnuts
Eggs	Vegetable oil	Filberts
Lard	Pecans	Soft margarine
	Olive Oil	Almonds
Plant Sources	Canola Oil	Mayonnaise
Cocoa butter (chocolates)	Stick margarine	Soybean oil
Coconut oil	Peanut oil	Corn oil
Palm kernel oil	Peanut butter	Sunflower oil
Palm oil	Cottonseed oil	Safflower oil
	Avocados	Sesame oil

Elevated blood cholesterol, which is caused by the consumption of saturated fat, clearly is an established risk factor for coronary artery disease (see Chapter 14). From a dietary point of view, the first line of therapy for elevated cholesterol is lowering saturated fat (including transfat) and cholesterol consumption. Unfortunately, the average adult in the U.S. consumes more than 400 mg of cholesterol — 33 percent more than the recommended maximum of 300 mg — every day. To put this in perspective, take note that the yolk of an average egg contains 215 mg of cholesterol. Egg whites, on the other hand, are cholesterol-free.

Use less salt and choose prepared foods with less salt

Although the American Heart Association recommends that adults consume daily less than 6 grams of salt (sodium chloride), or about 2,400 milligrams of sodium, the average adult in the U.S. consumes more than twice that much — 12 to 16 grams of salt per day (approximately 5 to 7 grams of sodium). That means the average person consumes about 2 or 3 teaspoons of salt daily rather than the recommended 1 teaspoon. Now, I know you don't sprinkle that much salt over your food at the table, but many prepared and convenience foods have high levels of sodium — take a glance at the labels. The same goes for restaurant offerings whether they're fast food or haute cuisine.

The major reason to limit salt/sodium intake has to do with its association with high blood pressure. In societies where less sodium is consumed, the incidence of high blood pressure is dramatically lower than it is in the U.S. If people with hypertension pay more attention to strict limitations on salt consumption and control their weight, many can manage blood pressure without medications.

Saturated fat alert

Saturated fat, often hidden, lies in wait for you. But when you know where to look for it, you can trim the amount that you consume without sacrificing good eating. Some of the places you can find saturated fat include

✔ **Visible fat on all meat and in chicken and turkey skin:** Trim whatever fat (and poultry skin) you can see.

✔ **Processed meats — hot dogs, salami, lunchmeat, and sausage:** These meats can derive 75 percent or more of their calories from saturated fat. Select fat-free products or put one slice of salami with sliced lean turkey for all the flavor but only a fourth of the fat.

✔ **Butterfat, present in cream and whole milk and products made with them:** Luxury ice cream is loaded. Select skim or 1 percent milk; low-fat or nonfat sour cream, cream cheese, and cottage cheese. Look for ice cream treats that are nonfat or lower fat.

✔ **Vegetable fats, such as palm oil and hydrogenated vegetable fats, present in prepared mixes and foods (cookies, bakery goods, cake mixes):** Check out the list of ingredients on the labels of the products you buy.

✔ **Fried and processed foods — those chips, that frozen dinner, or pizza:** Again check out the amount of fat listed on the label. If you must have those puff-a-pops, pick the one with the least fat/saturated fat.

Adding healthy zip to your food

Cutting fat, cholesterol, and salt doesn't necessarily mean cutting flavor. Keeping these five items on hand gives me plenty of ways to add some zip to food, while eating a low-fat and low-salt diet.

✔ **Vegetable and fruit salsas:** From party dips to dressings for salads or vegetables or sauces for fish, salsas are versatile. Find a good prepared salsa to keep on hand (watch out for too much sodium) and experiment with your own freshly made combinations.

✔ **Chilis:** Some like it hot! Supermarkets these days offer a good range of peppers hot and hotter. And for the pantry shelf, hundreds of hot sauces are available. You use so little that sodium usually isn't a problem. From the Caribbean to Asia and the entire globe in between, every style of cooking has creative uses for the pepper. It's a kick that won't hurt you.

✔ **Mustards:** Did you know hundreds of different mustards are on the market, ready for you to use? Mustards are a great substitute for traditional fats in dressing everything from sandwiches to entrees. Some can be pretty high in sodium (salt), but a little mustard goes a long way.

✔ **Balsamic (and other) vinegars:** A good balsamic vinegar is so nutty and sweet that many folks enjoy it alone as a salad dressing. Try the many specialty and flavored vinegars available to add a piquant touch to much more than just salads.

✔ **Fresh (or dried) herbs:** Dill, basil, cilantro, thyme, rosemary, oregano, chives . . . just the names make my mouth water. Supermarkets now carry a wider range of fresh herbs, and many of them are easy to grow, even as potted plants. After you taste what fresh basil can do for a tomato or pasta or what a rosemary sprig and lemon juice can do for a grilled fish filet or chicken breast, you'll be looking for more opportunities to use fresh herbs.

Choose beverages and foods to moderate your intake of sugars

Who doesn't like a little something sweet? Unfortunately, most Americans consume far too many *empty calories* (calories with no nutritional value) in the form of soft drinks, cookies, ice cream, candy, and other sweet treats. Think about these possible choices: One average candy bar or one half-cup serving of a premium ice cream contains about 275 to 300 calories (much of which is sugar and fat). For the same number of calories, you can eat two to three bananas, pears, or apples; or three to four peaches, apricots, or plums; an entire cantaloupe; a big wedge of watermelon; or a quart-and-a-half of strawberries. You no doubt get my drift. Plenty of good-for-you treats are available. Go ahead and enjoy the occasional ice cream or candy, but for everyday eating, think in terms of "more is less" — more fruit (more nutrition) is less caloric intake.

Look Mom, low cholesterol!

Dietary cholesterol, which is found exclusively in animal tissue, is more prevalent in eggs and organ meats. Here some tips for avoiding it.

Eggs. Most people know that eggs are high in cholesterol. One average egg yolk has 215 mg. But you can have your eggs and avoid cholesterol, too.

✔ Substitute two egg whites (0 mg cholesterol) for one whole egg in most any recipe in which the egg doesn't star.

✔ Use egg substitute or cholesterol-free egg products.

✔ For scrambled eggs/omelets, use one whole egg and one white instead of two whole.

✔ Use an egg substitute.

Organ meats. Liver, for instance, is just loaded with cholesterol. One 3-ounce slice of beef liver has 410 mg; one chicken liver has 125 mg. So if you like organ meats, save brains, sweetbreads, gizzards, hearts, and kidneys for a treat. If you hate liver, here's an excuse never to eat it again.

If you consume alcohol, do so in moderation

From a cardiovascular point of view, alcohol consumption is a complex issue. Moderate alcohol consumption actually has been shown to lower the risk of heart attack. Yet, alcohol also is loaded with calories and may, therefore, contribute to weight gain. Furthermore, excessive alcohol consumption actually carries with it the cardiovascular risk of increasing blood pressure and acting in adverse ways on the cardiac muscle itself.

The reason that moderate alcohol consumption may lower the risk of heart attack seems to come from two actions of alcohol. First, alcohol raises the HDL (the good cholesterol) level in the blood, and increased HDL is associated with decreased risk of heart disease. Second, some forms of alcoholic beverages impede blood clotting. Blood clotting is a dangerous process that contributes to heart attacks. Red wine, in particular, seems to impede blood clotting. (Red grape juice works, too.) Although the actual substances in red wine that contribute to this effect are not fully understood, a particular class of compounds known as *flavonoids* is thought to make a major contribution to decreased blood clotting. Flavonoids are found in the skins of grapes, which are left on longer in making red wine than white wine.

Moderate alcohol consumption generally is defined as one shot of distilled spirits or two glasses of wine or two beers on a daily basis. The most recent recommendations are no more than one alcoholic drink a day for a woman and no more than two for a man. Higher levels of alcohol consumption carry unacceptable health risks.

Grabbing more fruits, veggies, and grains

Fruits, vegetables, and grains seem to come in an almost endless variety. Eating more complex carbohydrates is easy and full of flavor. Do so by

✔ Getting whole grains at breakfast. Choose cereals, breads, and muffins made with whole grains (and not too much sugar).

✔ Choosing fruit for snacks and for dessert.

✔ Thinking fruit juice rather than soft drink for that afternoon thirst-quencher/pick-me-up.

✔ Featuring vegetables, whole-grain pastas, and grains instead of meat at dinner. Avoid fatty or cream sauces and gravies.

✔ Avoiding empty sugar carbohydrates in candy and snacks.

✔ Trying one new vegetable or fruit or a new way of preparing them once a week.

✔ Choosing the bread and rejecting the spread. Bread usually does not have too many calories, but the butter, oil, or jam you put on it probably does.

Don't consume more calories than you need to maintain your best body weight

Obesity is a major risk factor for a variety of health consequences, but particularly for heart disease. About 75 percent of all mortality associated with obesity comes from the increased risk of heart disease. Although decreased consumption of fat calories decreases the risk of obesity, all calories from any source do count. The reason so many Americans are overweight is that they consume too many calories, period. Most Americans also get too little physical activity. Physical activity, as I discuss in Chapter 21, helps you maintain lean muscle mass, burn more calories, and enhance cardiac health.

Making Heart-Healthy Eating Part of Your Lifestyle

Whether you've tried and failed to develop healthy eating habits or are trying for the first time, the wealth of nutrition information available can be overwhelming. Start simple, with the three key rules and the simple guidelines that follow. Healthy eating doesn't require an advanced degree or complicated math that leaves you little time to actually eat. Modifying your diet without devoting your life to percentages and fat grams is not only possible, it's simple and tasty. Believe it or not, you can even dine out without falling off the wagon.

Slacking off the salt

Four easy steps can significantly lower the amount of salt in your diet:

✔ Never salting food without first tasting it

✔ Increasing your intake of fruits and vegetables and natural products that have minimal or no salt in them

✔ Taking the saltshaker off the table

✔ Cutting down on processed foods and "fast" foods that usually are loaded with salt

If you're a snack addict, look for one of the numerous low-fat and reduced-salt products, such as reduced-salt baked corn chips, pretzels, or potato chips that now are on the market.

Checking out three key rules for healthy eating

Sometimes the most important principles for healthy eating are the simplest ones, and yet they're often ignored. If your head is whirling with the guidelines I just discussed, here are just three simple heart-healthy practices that you can adopt immediately to make an enormous difference.

Rule No. 1: Eat a healthy, low-fat breakfast

The well-respected nutrition writer Jane Brody once was asked the most important nutritional practice that she had learned in her 25-year career. Her response: "Eat like a king for breakfast, a prince for lunch, and a pauper for supper." Unfortunately, many people do exactly the reverse. The health and nutrition reasons for consuming a good, low-fat breakfast are numerous. Here are just a few.

✔ Breakfast skippers tend to gain weight. Why? They tend to fill that mid-morning hungry feeling with a sweet or salty caloric snack.

✔ Matching calorie consumption with calorie expenditure is important. Consuming more of your calories in the morning gets you ready to face the demands of an active day. Whenever you eat most of your calories at night and then go to bed, your body thinks it's time to store those calories, and that contributes to weight gain.

✔ Breakfast is a great time for consuming fiber. Many people get up to 25 percent of their daily fiber at breakfast. With so many high-fiber breakfast cereals now available, increasing fiber consumption is easy, and better yet, it lowers your risk of heart disease.

✔ Breakfast is a great time for consuming fruits and vegetables. Pour yourself a tall glass of orange juice and put a sliced banana on your cereal, and you're 40 percent of the way to the recommended daily minimum of five servings of fruits and vegetables a day.

What's the perfect breakfast? A bowl of whole-grain cereal (whole grain oat cereal probably is the best, because the soluble fiber further lowers cholesterol) is hard to top, especially when you eat it with some sliced fruit, a glass of orange juice, a piece of whole-grain toast, and a cup of coffee or tea, all with skim milk. You say you prefer grapefruit, prune, or tomato juice, and low-fat oat-bran muffins for variety? That's great. You've got the general idea.

Rule No. 2: Eat at least five servings of fruits and vegetables every day

I can't emphasize the importance of this rule enough. Yes, it's the first guideline above. Fruits and vegetables give you loads of important nutrients, they're typically low in calories and fat (skip the cheese sauce, please), and they generally keep you feeling full and satisfied in a way that sugary or salty snacks don't.

Rule No. 3: Drink pure water

Folks tend to neglect the natural and healthful practice of drinking pure water. Instead, they substitute beverages that contain sugar, caffeine, or fat (milkshakes!). Caffeine and fat may increase blood pressure or increase the risk of heart disease. Empty sugar calories can lead to overconsumption of calories and weight gain.

Getting protein aplenty

The average American eats much more protein than necessary — or optimal — for good health. Most of this protein is consumed in the form of meat. Although eating a high-protein diet can help with short-term weight loss, you may end up paying a significant price. High-protein diets usually are also high in fat and may increase cholesterol. Consuming an adequate amount of protein doesn't take much effort:

✔ Eating two 2- to 3-oz servings of fish, lean meat, or poultry provides an adequate daily protein intake.

✔ Eating one egg or two egg whites provides protein equal to one ounce of meat or fish.

✔ Enjoying smaller portions of meat in combination main dishes such as pasta, stir-fries, or casseroles cuts back on protein consumption — just remember to avoid high fat.

✔ Adding tofu (soybean curd) to stir-fries and casseroles provides good protein with relatively low fat.

✔ Choosing bean dishes, particularly combos such as beans and rice or beans and whole-grain pasta, gives you a good source of protein and fiber.

What's a serving?

When scientists, registered dietitians, and food pyramid guides talk about servings, the quantities they mean may surprise most folks. A serving is probably much smaller than you think. Here are some of the typical amounts they have in mind for one serving.

Grain products 1 slice of bread

½ cup dry cereal

½ cup cooked rice, pasta, or cereal (like oatmeal)

Vegetables 1 cup raw leafy vegetables (lettuce, cabbage)

½ cup cooked vegetable

6 ounces vegetable juice

Fruits 1 medium fruit (apple, pear, orange)

¼ cup dried fruit

½ cup fresh, frozen, or canned-in-juice (not syrup) fruit

A serving of some fruits, such as strawberries or watermelon, can be a cup or more.

6 ounces fruit juice

Dairy products 1 cup skim or 1 percent milk

1 cup nonfat or low-fat yogurt or nonfat cottage cheese

1 ounce cheese (about 1-inch cube of cheddar, Monterey Jack, or Swiss)

Meat, poultry, fish 2 to 3 ounces cooked

Nuts, seeds 1½ ounces/⅓ cup nuts (peanuts, pecans, walnuts, cashews)

2 tablespoons seeds (sunflower, pumpkin)

Considering special issues in nutrition

Although low-fat, low-cholesterol eating is the cornerstone for heart-healthy nutrition, some additional tidbits on sound practices and some controversies can help you build on this solid, nutritional core.

✔ **Whole-grain oats:** Careful studies show that eating adequate amounts of whole-grain oats can further reduce cholesterol up to 5 percent to 6 percent over and above cholesterol reduction achieved from low-fat nutrition. That means for every 1 percent reduction in cholesterol, you get a 2 percent decrease in the likelihood of coronary artery disease. The amount of oats needed to achieve these benefits can be obtained in one good-sized bowl of Cheerios or similar oat cereal every day.

✔ **Fish:** Recent studies show that people who consume fish at least once a week lower their incidence of sudden death from cardiac disease. So that's just one more reason to eat fish — one of the most complete and healthy foods you can eat. It is a great source of protein and is low in saturated fats.

Shellfish (shrimp, lobster, oysters, clams, and so on), on the other hand, contains a lot of cholesterol, but because it has virtually no saturated fat, it certainly can be included in a heart-healthy diet.

✔ **Butter versus margarine:** For years, cardiologists advised people to limit their intake of butter and instead choose margarine, particularly soft margarine. Then, in 1994, a number of articles, including one from the Harvard School of Public Health, suggested that the transfats (hydrogenated or partially hydrogenated oils) found in margarine were worse for both cholesterol and LDL than butter. Of course, people screamed that once again the experts had misled them. My advice on this one is to limit your intake of butter and margarine. As I've already said, drizzling a little olive oil, with its beneficial monounsaturated fats, on your bread is a much better choice than either margarine or butter. If you choose margarine, pick one of the several products now formulated without transfats.

✔ **Nutrition for athletes and physically active people:** Sometimes athletes and physically active people think that they need to eat special diets to meet the demands of their physical activity. (Certain advertisements do their best to push this idea while hyping their products.) But the nutritional needs of highly active or athletic people change in only one way; they can consume a few more calories without weight gain because they're burning more calories. Sound nutrition for physically active people is based on the same principles that I've already described for heart-healthy nutrition for nonactive people.

✔ **Fad diets:** Unfortunately, people who are trying to lose weight often get sucked into following fad diets. Recent popular diets include those that advocate increasing the amount of protein in the diet, lowering carbohydrate intake, or increasing the amount of fat in the diet. Although these diets have achieved a certain popularity for weight loss, they're not wise from a cardiovascular standpoint. When used for more than short-term weight loss (and perhaps even then), these approaches can significantly raise your cholesterol.

Other fad diets may promote supposedly scientific practices (often food combinations) that make your body burn fat more rapidly in heretofore unknown or secret ways. Unfortunately, regardless of their claims, most of these diets have no basis in scientific fact. More important, however, any short-term weight loss you achieve usually cannot be sustained nor can health benefits be realized, because the diets don't foster balanced, healthy approaches to eating for the long-term.

Counting ketchup as a vegetable? Tips for heart-healthy dining out

Eat at some fast food joints on a regular basis, and you'd certainly have to count ketchup as a vegetable to have any hope of eating your daily five. And don't even think about avoiding excess fat! But dining out need not be so fraught with peril for your healthy eating goals. If you keep these simple tips in mind, you can eat out, eat well, and eat right.

- ✔ **Select a restaurant that can help you stay on plan.** Whether you're headed out for fine dining or fast food (or anything in between), you can choose a restaurant that helps you meet your goals. For example, a sandwich shop where you can select lean ingredients and fixings may be a better choice than a place that offers only burgers and fries. The same sort of distinctions also can apply at better restaurants.

- ✔ **Order wisely to make the menu work for you.** Almost every restaurant offers items and/or methods of preparation that you can enjoy with a cheerful heart. Make the menu work for you with wise selections:

    - Broiled, baked, or roasted rather than fried

    - Vegetable or clear sauces rather than butter or cream sauces

    - Steamed rather than creamed or fried veggies

    - Dressing on the side for your salad

- ✔ **Practice portion control.** "Bigger is better" seems to be the catchphrase for portions at many restaurants. When presented with a plate heaped with enough for two or three, resist temptation — eat what you need, and take the rest home to Fido, or leave it. If the restaurant deserves a repeat visit, maybe you can share that great dish with a friend. You can also order an appetizer as an entree or seek restaurants that specialize in small-plate offerings.

- ✔ **Enjoy the occasional blowout.** Remember that Greek tyrant Procrustes who chopped off visitors to fit his guest bed? That isn't what heart-healthy eating is about. If a juicy steak with all the trimmings or a classic French dinner with great wines is your idea of the proper way to cele-brate, *bon appetit!* Healthy eating is about overall moderation and bal-ance. Only one caution: If your cardiologist has told you to avoid certain practices, pay close attention.

Managing your weight with heart-healthy eating

If you choose the foods you eat and preparation methods to promote heart health, you'll also be adopting practices that can help you lose weight (if you need to) and manage your weight at healthy levels for the rest of your life. An effective weight-loss plan based on the guidelines for heart-healthy nutrition also will feature a planned reduction in calories consumed and a planned increase in physical activity — the basis of any long-term weight management plan.

As you work to adopt heart-healthy nutrition and plan to lose weight, you may want to get some expert help. Your cardiologist may recommend a professional dietitian, or you may need to find one yourself.

Believe it or not, anybody can call themselves a *nutritionist,* regardless of their training or expertise. For professional help in planning new ways of eating, I recommend that you consult a registered dietitian (RD). The RD after that professional's name means that he or she has earned a professional degree (or degrees) in nutrition and has successfully completed the national credentialing exam and other qualifications set by the Commission on Dietetic Registration of the American Dietetics Association (ADA). You can reach the Nationwide Nutrition Network, the ADA's referral service, at 800-366-1655.

Incorporating other components of a healthy lifestyle

Nutrition is of great importance to a heart-healthy lifestyle, but please remember that it is not a magic bullet. When you pay attention to sound nutritional practices and combine them with managing your weight and incorporating regular physical activity in your life, you achieve three of the most important pillars of daily lifestyle habits and actions that contribute to an overall heart-healthy lifestyle.

Checking out two heart-healthy diets

For a long time, doctors and dietitians have known that residents of the countries around the Mediterranean Sea seem to have a lower incidence of heart disease than is the case in most other countries. Many argue that the so-called *Mediterranean Diet,* which is high in monounsaturated fats (largely from olive oil), grains and vegetables, makes a major contribution to the low incidence of heart disease in this region. Monounsaturated fats seem to raise the HDL (the good cholesterol) but not total cholesterol. The American Heart Association and the American Dietetic Association have increasingly used Mediterranean-styled diets as recommendations for lowering your risk of chronic disease. One downside of any oil, however, is that it's loaded with calories. Just remember to use oil in moderation.

Although the *DASH Diet* was designed as part of a research study that tested the effect of dietary patterns on preventing and lowering high blood pressure, it offers an excellent approach for general heart health. DASH stands for Dietary Approaches to Stop Hypertension, an eating plan that reduces total and saturated fat intake and emphasizes fruits, vegetables, and low-fat dairy foods. It also limits your intake of sweets. Read all about the DASH Diet on the DASH page (nhlbi.nih.gov/health/public/heart/hbp/dash) of the Web site of The National Heart, Lung, and Blood Institute (NHLBI), the study's sponsor. Among other resources, you can download a booklet with menus or you can obtain one by writing to the NHLBI Information Center, P.O. Box 30105, Bethesda, MD 20824-0105.

Chapter 21

Getting It in Gear: Physical Activity and Exercise for Heart Health

---

---

*T*he good news is that physical activity not only helps prevent heart disease, but it also plays an important role in the therapy for people who have various cardiac conditions. The principles that I discuss in this chapter are appropriate for both situations, but I want to emphasize clearly that if you have existing heart disease, you must carefully discuss physical activity with your personal physician, so that together you can plan an activity program that's appropriate for you and your particular condition. With that caution in mind, physical activity offers many health benefits for everyone.

Understanding Physical Activity and What It Can Do for Heart Health

Literally hundreds of scientific and medical studies document the cardiac benefits of regular exercise. These studies recently were summarized in the *Surgeon General's Report on Physical Activity and Health*. By the same token, inactivity poses a serious risk of developing heart disease. In one major summary study combining the results of 43 previous studies, for example, scientists from the Centers for Disease Control (CDC) conclude that inactive people double their risk of heart disease when compared with active people. By CDC criteria, more than 60 percent of the adult population in the United States falls into the *inactive* category. It's time to get off the couch.

Recognizing the difference between physical activity and exercise

Once when I was giving a speech about the importance of regular physical activity for heart health, a woman stood up and said, "That may be important, but I had my fill of wearing gym shorts back in grade school. I'll never do it again!"

This woman was expressing the classic confusion between exercise and physical activity. Although considerable overlap exists between the two, they are not exactly the same.

- ✔ **Physical activity** is a much broader concept than exercise and can be defined as any muscular movement that utilizes energy. Sitting on your couch, for example, is not physical activity. Getting your butt off of that couch is!

- ✔ **Exercise** is a *type* of physical activity that typically is defined more narrowly as a planned and structured activity where bodily movements are repeated to achieve various aspects of fitness. Most people usually think of exercise as activities such as aerobic dance, jogging, or swimming laps.

Drawing a distinction between physical activity and exercise may seem like nit-picking, but the distinction is important from a practical standpoint. Many people don't realize that simply getting out of their easy chairs and raking the leaves on a brisk autumn day or spending an hour gardening classifies as physical activity and that such physical activity during a lifetime has been shown to lower the risk of heart disease.

Identifying the benefits of physical activity

Getting regular physical activity can help you

- ✔ Lower your risk of heart disease
- ✔ Improve your quality of life
- ✔ Reduce anxiety and tension and elevate your mood

✔ Improve your risk factors for other diseases such as cancer and diabetes

✔ Achieve and maintain a healthy body weight

And getting plenty of physical activity provides more specific benefits for heart health.

If you want to prevent heart disease

Even if you feel fine and fit or even if your doctor gave you the thumbs up at your last checkup, you can experience several positive changes after just two or three months of regular physical activity.

✔ Tasks that previously made you short of breath are easier to perform.

✔ Your heart rate when you're resting is lower. Because a more efficient heart pumps more blood on each beat, it requires fewer beats per minute to supply your body with oxygen when you're simply sitting still. Some people believe that this lower heart rate is one of the reasons why fit people live longer. The famous cardiologist Dr. Paul Dudley White, who was former President Dwight Eisenhower's physician, once said, "The heart is programmed at birth for a certain number of beats. I'd rather take mine at 50 beats per minute than 75!"

✔ Your heart is a stronger muscle. During a lifetime of moderate physical activity, the heart, as a muscle, maintains better condition than the heart of someone who remains or becomes inactive.

✔ The coronary arteries, which supply blood to the heart, are more likely to stay large and relatively clean in individuals who exercise on a regular basis. Remember that clean coronary arteries prevent heart attacks (see Chapter 3).

If you have heart disease

Whether you have a condition like high blood pressure that's a risk factor for heart disease, you have symptoms of coronary artery disease (CAD) like angina, or you've experienced a heart attack, regular physical activity can help you achieve better health. Depending on your current condition, some modifications may be necessary.

✔ **If you have high blood pressure (hypertension):** (See also Chapter 13.) Regular physical activity not only reduces the risk of developing hypertension, but also is effective as a treatment for hypertension. The most significant change your physician typically makes in any moderate physical activity is to require that you reduce your level of exertion about 10 percent below that of people who do not have high blood pressure.

✔ **If you have coronary artery disease (CAD):** Physical activity programs can help people with CAD increase their ability to perform activities of daily life and lower their risk of having additional problems with CAD. If you have angina (chest pain), your physician will instruct you to conduct your physical activity program at least 15 beats per minute below the level at which you experience chest pain.

✔ **If you've had a heart attack:** (See also Chapter 5.) If you've suffered a heart attack, you need to begin your program of physical activity in a supervised cardiac rehabilitation program under the guidance of a trained cardiologist (see also Chapter 18). Physical activity can help strengthen your damaged heart and help it function more efficiently, and a fit body requires less work from the heart. Physical activity also helps prevent a second heart event by helping you reduce cholesterol levels, control high blood pressure, control diabetes, and manage weight, all of which contribute to heart disease.

✔ **If you have heart failure:** (See also Chapter 7.) In the normal heart, approximately 70 percent to 80 percent of the blood that is returned to the heart is pumped out with each beat. In an individual who has heart failure, less than 40 percent, and in some instances as low as 15 percent to 20 percent, of the blood that is returned to the heart is pumped out with each beat. If you have heart failure, appropriate lower-intensity physical activity can help you to increase the efficiency of your muscles so that they require less blood flow from the heart.

If you are older

Physical activity has been shown to be beneficial for people of all ages. If you reach the age of 65, you have an 80 percent chance of reaching the age of 80! Reducing your risk of heart disease and contributing factors such as high cholesterol, high blood pressure, and diabetes is important at any age, and keeping the heart and muscles in tune is particularly important for older individuals.

Knowing How Much Physical Activity Is Enough

Many people are confused about how much physical activity is required to lower their risk of heart disease or otherwise help them manage a heart condition. They also wonder how hard they need to work at it. Recent guidelines from the Centers for Disease Control (CDC) and the American College of Sports Medicine (ACSM) recommend that every adult try to accumulate at least 30 minutes of moderate-intensity physical activity on most if not all days. Depending upon your actual state of physical fitness and heart health, your physician can help you determine what's appropriate for you. But the two key concepts — *accumulating activity* and *moderate intensity* — apply to everyone.

Cashing in on the other benefits of physical activity

Although this chapter focuses largely on the cardiovascular benefits of regular physical activity, the simple decision to be physically active confers many other health benefits. Here are a few:

✔ **Decreasing cancer risks:** Rapidly accumulating strong evidence suggests that regular physical activity cuts down on your risk of cancer. In particular, the risk for cancers that seem to have a hormonal component, such as breast cancer in women and prostate cancer in men, seems to be lowered by regular physical activity. Studies also show that the risk of colon cancer also decreases in people who are physically active. A recent study from Stanford University indicated that women who are physically active for two to four hours per week decrease their risk of breast cancer by 50 percent.

✔ **Preventing diabetes:** Physical activity also is a great way of lowering your risk of diabetes. Studies show that physically active people reduce their risks of adult onset diabetes between 24 percent and 100 percent.

✔ **Achieving and maintaining a healthy body weight:** People who are inactive are much more likely to gain weight during their lives than people who are physically active. The expenditure of calories on a regular basis also tends to preserve lean muscle mass and make you capable of increased levels of functioning throughout your life.

✔ **Improving mental and emotional states:** Numerous studies show that physical activity reduces anxiety and tension and can improve mood and decrease the likelihood of depression.

Accumulating activity

Those short bursts of physical activity that you perform each day add up or *accumulate* to provide you with the same benefit as going to the gym for 30 minutes (an impossibly short trip). So look for ways to accumulate physical activity in your daily life. Take the stairs instead of the elevator. Park farther away from the store and walk to your destination. Take a simple fitness walk for ten minutes at lunchtime. All those activities count.

Using moderate intensity

Moderate intensity activities provide a level of exertion that is between light and heavy. In other words, the type of activity that you choose needs to be intense enough so that you know you're exerting yourself, but not so intense that you're out of breath with sweat running down your brow.

Here are examples of moderate activity that you can accumulate in various increments of time:

- ✔ Bowling
- ✔ Cleaning
- ✔ Gardening
- ✔ Horseback riding
- ✔ Leisurely cycling
- ✔ Mopping
- ✔ Mowing the lawn
- ✔ No-load hiking
- ✔ Painting walls

- ✔ Raking the leaves
- ✔ Recreational tennis
- ✔ Shooting baskets
- ✔ Slow swimming
- ✔ Sweeping
- ✔ Table tennis
- ✔ Vacuuming
- ✔ Walking
- ✔ Washing the car

I'll never forget when my laboratory first started performing walking research. Jay Leno joked on *The Tonight Show,* "Now they tell us that walking is good for us — the next thing they'll be saying is that sitting is good for us!" Although the audience laughed, Leno actually was stating a common myth that you need to exert yourself to a high level to achieve any cardiac benefits. Research clearly shows that walking is adequate for achieving almost all cardiac benefits; moreover, walking (and other regular, moderate-intensity activities) can significantly lower your risk of developing heart disease or help you live well with it.

Thinking no pain, no gain? No way!

Many people mistakenly think that exercise needs to be painful to be beneficial. Nothing could be farther from the truth, particularly when you have heart disease. In fact, if exercise is painful, it probably isn't good for anyone. Furthermore, for heart patients, pain, particularly chest pain, typically is a warning sign that you're exerting yourself too hard. Slow down.

Easing on down the road — into a great start

If you charge into exercise, you'll wear yourself out at best and injure yourself at worst (particularly if you have a heart problem). Here are four basic ways to make sure that you stay within the *moderate* exertion zone — and stay with it.

✔ **Take the talk test.** Make sure that you can carry on a normal conversation with a companion while you're engaged in a bout of physical activity.

✔ **Check out your perceived exertion.** Pay attention to your body. Ask yourself, "Am I exerting myself at a moderate level or am I actually exerting myself at a light level or heavy level?" Be honest with yourself. (Nobody but you is going to blab.) Research shows that by using this subjective gauge, most people can accurately determine whether they're working at a moderate intensity level of exertion. If you have high blood pressure, talk to your doctor about appropriate intensity levels. Individuals with high blood pressure or angina, for instance, usually need to work at light-moderate or lower-intensity levels.

✔ **Take your pulse.** With a little practice, you can find your pulse on the thumb side of the inside of the wrist. Count your pulse for ten seconds and then multiply by six to find out your heart rate in beats per minute during exertion. Moderate exertion for a healthy individual takes place between 60 percent and 70 percent of your predicted maximum heart rate. For individuals with high blood pressure or a heart condition, moderate exertion takes place at lower percentages of maximum exertion, so ask your physician for specific instructions.

To estimate your maximum heart rate, subtract your age in years from 220 beats per minute. Thus, for a 40-year-old individual, the predicted maximum heart rate is 220 beats minus 40 beats — 180 beats per minute. The moderate exertion level of 60 percent to 70 percent of 180 beats equals 108 to 126 beats per minute.

✔ **Use a heart-rate monitor.** You can find inexpensive heart-rate monitors on the market that accurately keep track of your heartbeat during exercise and take the hassle out of accurately determining your exertion level. I particularly recommend the use of a heart-rate monitor if you have high blood pressure or any type of heart disease, or if you've experienced a heart attack.

Getting Started the Right Way

Most people have trouble getting started with regular activity or exercise for one simple reason: They make it too complex. Ask yourself these three questions to increase your chance of selecting the right activity program. And then answer them honestly. (No daydreams of making the next Olympic team.)

✔ What do I like to do?

✔ What is convenient for me?

✔ What have I successfully done in the past?

For many people, the answer to these questions is walking. For others (depending on heart health, too), the physical activity of choice may be swimming, jogging, tai chi, aerobic dance, yoga, in-line skating, or other forms of regular exertion.

Avoid the deadly home-gym syndrome. You have an acute case of home-gym syndrome the first time that you buy a piece of exercise equipment and take it home only to hang clothes on it. You have a chronic case of home-gym syndrome when you buy the second piece of home fitness equipment and now have a matched pair of expensive clothes racks.

Don't get me wrong . . . I'm not against fitness equipment. In fact, I have three or four pieces of home fitness equipment in both of my workout areas. But be realistic and choose forms of exercise that are simple, enjoyable, and convenient.

Choosing the best activity for you

People often ask me what is the best activity or exercise to promote heart health and general fitness. My answer never changes: It is the form of exercise that you will do! Look at *all* the things you like to do, because somewhere in that list is an activity that will get you started.

Starting your program with aerobic exercise

Every beginning exerciser needs to build his or her program around a core of what are called *aerobic* exercises. *Aerobic* literally means "in the presence of air." So aerobic exercises are those that require your muscles to burn more oxygen and you to breathe faster. Hard-working, air-hungry muscles demand more oxygen-rich blood from the heart. The heart in turn works a little harder and grows stronger. In this way, aerobic exercise helps lower the risk of heart disease. Although you work at lower levels of intensity when you already have heart disease, aerobic activity still will be the foundation of your activity program.

Mixing and matching activities

Many different kinds of aerobic activities and exercises exist. All of them are good for the heart. Pick the ones that you think may be most convenient for you, or, better yet, mix and match. I also need to emphasize that daily forms of physical activity, such as leaf raking, lawn work, gardening, even brisk housework, all qualify as *moderate* physical activity and all are equally beneficial for the heart. Make them part of your overall plan.

What about strength training?

Recently, considerable attention has been paid to the health benefits of strength training. Although strength training has multiple overall benefits, it should not be the core exercise for people who want to prevent heart disease or, in particular, who already have heart disease.

Virtually all medical literature supporting the link between exercise and preventing heart disease comes from studies of aerobic exercise. In fact, strength training may be contraindicated in patients who already have coronary artery disease (CAD) or high blood pressure. The problem with strength training in people with these problems is that it can cause dramatic increases in blood pressure. These increases in blood pressure, in turn, cause the heart to work harder, which can pose a particular problem for people who already have narrowing of the coronary arteries. Likewise, people who have hypertension also can experience significant and even dangerous increases in their blood pressure if they do any heavy lifting during strength training.

Nonetheless, strength training can be useful in the reduction of your risk of heart disease or in treatment of heart disease. Strength training can benefit heart patients by increasing the efficiency of their muscles, thus enabling them to carry out either leisure-time or work activities at a lower percentage of their maximal capacity. Regular strength training also can help prevent weight gain, which is of significant benefit for patients with heart disease.

If you already have heart disease and want to start strength training, or if you want to use strength training to lower your risk of heart disease, the best advice is to find a skilled health professional with knowledge and background in cardiac rehabilitation. This person can help you establish the best routine for you. These routines typically are based on high-repetition, low-weight strength training. This approach enables your muscles to become more efficient without risking the danger of dramatic elevations in blood pressure.

Here are some aerobic activities you might enjoy:

- Walking
- Cross-country skiing
- Cycling, outdoors
- Cycling, stationary
- Dancing, jazz, modern, tap
- In-line skating
- Aerobic dance
- Rowing
- Running/jogging
- Stair climbing
- Swimming

Involving your physician

Preventing or managing heart disease requires teamwork. As I said earlier, let your doctor know of your desire to participate in a program of regular physical activity and seek his or her guidance. Most doctors welcome the opportunity to talk about lifestyle measures with you and can help you fine-tune your physical activity program to account for your unique personal circumstances such as current medications, current level of physical activity, and current physical conditions, including existing heart disease. You may consider having an exercise tolerance test before starting to exercise.

If you already have any heart condition, taking an exercise tolerance test prior to starting a program of physical activity is important. Talk to your physician about it. In addition, older people, people who have one or more risk factors for heart disease (see Chapter 3), and people who have been inactive also may benefit from such testing. The American Heart Association and the American College of Sports Medicine recommend that men older than the age of 50 and women older than the age of 55 who've lived previously sedentary lifestyles have a physician-supervised exercise tolerance test before starting a new exercise program.

Developing a personal plan for physical activity

When it comes to sticking with physical activity long term, people usually falter on simple issues rather than complex issues. In addition to choosing an activity (or activities) that is enjoyable, convenient, and with which you've been successful in the past, you must remember that achieving the goal of a healthier heart through physical activity is a race that is won by the tortoise and not the hare.

Adopting the following watch words can help you plan your personal program. In fact, you may even want to post them on your mirror or tape them to your sweatband.

- ✔ Start slow.
- ✔ Progress slowly.
- ✔ Use common sense to avoid dangerous symptoms.
- ✔ When in doubt, ask your doc. (Even if you think your question is silly, the risk of embarrassment is much less harmful than going down with a heart attack or, worse yet, sudden death.)

If you've previously been inactive, starting out at a low level of moderate intensity, such as walking five minutes per day, represents a good beginning. After you're comfortable with that level of exertion, you can increase it slowly. Try building up your walk or other activity by approximately one minute per week until you reach 30 minutes on most, if not all, days.

Gearing up for success

One of the easiest ways to increase the likelihood that you'll stick with your exercise program is obtaining proper gear. In the case of walking or running, this can be very simple. The most important gear for walkers and runners is proper footwear and clothing.

You can get good advice about walking or running shoes appropriate for your level of fitness, the terrain that you walk or run on, and climatic conditions in which you exercise at any good shoe store. Finding proper, well-fitting footwear increases your comfort during your walk or run and thereby encourages you to stick with your program. One tip for buying walking or running shoes is to do so during the afternoon because your feet tend to swell a little bit during the day, and you get a better fit when you try them on in the afternoon.

Like shoes, clothing can enhance your workouts when it fits you properly and keeps out the elements. Most regular exercisers understand the value of *layering* their exercise clothing. Select good athletic clothes all the way from running or walking shorts and T-shirts on up to a jogging or walking suit. If you exercise in cold, rainy, or snowy weather, some of the newer products such as water-resistant running suits can increase the likelihood that you'll exercise during foul weather. A hat and gloves also are important and often neglected aspects of athletic clothing.

Of course, don't leave your common sense at home! If you have any symptoms such as chest discomfort during a walk, you need to slow down or stop and discuss the symptom at the earliest possible time with your doctor. Remember that the most important heart benefits from regular physical activity accrue to individuals who find ways of remaining physically active throughout their lives.

Walking Your Way to a Healthier Heart

Patients often ask me what exercise I recommend for heart health. My enthusiastic answer never changes — walking! Yes, walking — that simple skill you've been competent in since you were a year old. Most people, however, underestimate the power of regular fitness walking. In fact, many 50- and 60-year-olds enrolled in the walking studies at my research laboratory assert that "walking would only be good for someone like my parents" — who must be in their 80s or 90s! Of course, walking is good for their parents, but it's also good for them.

Hooking a fish tale with a moral

Talking about cardiovascular health to people who expect it to mean Olympic-level training reminds me of two sofa jockeys who decided to go on a weekend fishing trip. After they packed up all their camping gear and fishing tackle, one man also packed his running shoes, thinking he might get back into a little physical activity. Well, as the men were tramping across a meadow on the way to their campsite, a ferocious grizzly bear suddenly broke into the open on the far side of the meadow and started running toward them. They froze with terror. Then one man began to run for the nearest tree. The other, however, dropped his pack, grabbed his running shoes, and calmly began lacing them up. His fleeing companion yelled over his shoulder, "You're the stupidest man I ever met. No one can outrun a grizzly bear!" "Who said anything about the bear, my friend?" the first replied, rising to his feet. "I simply intend to outrun you!"

What's the point? Most people think that they need to outrun the ferocious grizzly bears of their inactive past (or even their poor heart health), when all they really need to do to get most of the cardiovascular benefits from exercise is to outrun (or *outwalk* — as I hope to convince you) their previously sedentary selves. This maxim is doubly true for anyone with heart disease.

Considering why walking is the best heart-healthy exercise

Extensive research conducted by my laboratory and others demonstrates some simple facts about walking.

- ✔ Virtually everyone can get aerobic benefit from walking. Walking is particularly suitable for patients with a variety of heart conditions because the intensity is extremely flexible.

- ✔ Walking is usually the simplest and most convenient form of physical activity for the vast majority of people.

- ✔ Walking is simple — as easy as putting one foot in front of the other, opening your front door, and setting off down the road.

- ✔ Most of the research that shows that regular physical activity lowers the risk of heart disease has focused on walking.

- ✔ For most people, I recommend walking as the best form of regular exercise to lower the risk of cardiovascular disease — and so do 90 percent of my fellow physicians.

Still need more convincing? The number of fitness walkers in the United States is three times the number of joggers. Currently, inactive individuals who say they want to start an exercise program choose walking 6 times as frequently as jogging and 18 times more often than aerobic dance.

If you prefer a different form of physical activity and/or aerobic exercise, however, don't be dismayed. Almost everything I say about walking also applies to other forms of aerobic exercise. All aerobic activities are equally good in terms of their cardiovascular benefits.

Walking for weight management

Walking is an excellent adjunct to a program for managing your weight properly. Walking and other forms of physical activity not only burn calories but also help maintain a lower weight over the long haul.

Walking consistently can make an enormous difference in terms of weight control. For example, if you weigh 175 pounds and walk two miles every day, you can lose up to 20 pounds in one year as long as you don't increase your caloric intake.

Most people underestimate how many calories you can burn during a walking session. Table 21-1 shows how many calories you burn per mile based on your walking pace and body weight.

Table 21-1		Caloric Cost of Walking (Calories/Mile)					
Walking Pace		*Body Weight*					
(mph)	*(min/mile)*	*100*	*125*	*150*	*175*	*200*	*225*
		Calories Burned					
2.0	30	60	75	90	105	120	136
2.2	27	58	72	87	101	116	130
2.4	25	56	70	84	98	113	127
2.7	22	53	66	79	92	105	118
3.0	20	53	66	79	92	105	118
3.3	18	53	67	79	92	105	118
3.5	17	54	67	81	94	108	121
3.75	16	56	69	83	97	111	125
4.0	15	58	73	87	102	116	131
4.3	14	62	77	92	108	123	139

Sticking with It through the Long Haul

Following these five tips can help you stick with your program of accumulating moderate-intensity activities.

- ✔ **Set a time and place.** Most people find that routines are helpful, so try to establish at least one time and place for physical activity each day. How about walking the dog in the morning, or taking a ten-minute, mind-clearing walk at lunch?

- ✔ **Be prepared.** Always be on the lookout for unexpected opportunities to insert a little activity into the nooks and crannies of your life. Adopt a mind-set that emphasizes more physical activity.

- ✔ **Include family and friends.** Undertaking activities with family and friends makes them more social and enjoyable. This practice also increases the likelihood that you'll carve out time for physical activity each day.

- ✔ **Have fun.** If your activity isn't fun, you aren't going to do it. Choose things that you look forward to doing.

- ✔ **Prioritize.** If you don't make physical activity a priority, you're highly unlikely to stay with it day in and day out, week in and week out, month in and month out.

Making Sure You Don't Overdo It

Too much of a good thing is not, as Mae West would have you believe, "marvelous." When it comes to exercise, too much can be hard on your heart and your health. Don't think that's an excuse not to exercise; it's simply a warning that you need to take it slow and keep close tabs on how you feel during and after activity.

Recognizing six signs of overexercising

When starting an exercise program, many people don't realize how easy it is to overexercise. Watch out for these warning signals:

- ✔ **Difficulty finishing:** If you can't complete your exercise program with energy to spare, decrease your walking pace and/or your distance.

- ✔ **Inability to carry on a normal conversation while walking:** If you can't talk normally while you exercise, you're going too fast. Slow down!

- ✔ **Faintness or nausea after exercising:** If your walking is too intense or you stop walking too abruptly, you can feel faint. This happens because increased blood flow to your legs when you're walking may cause blood to pool temporarily in the veins, making it difficult for the heart to maintain an adequate output. Decrease your walking pace and increase the amount of time you spend cooling down. If you nonetheless feel faint again, see your doctor.

✔ **Chronic fatigue:** If during the remainder of the day or evening after exercise you feel tired rather than stimulated, you're exercising too hard. If you feel fatigued or experience chest pain after exercise, decrease the pace and/or distance of your workout. Seeing your doctor also is a good idea.

✔ **Sleeplessness:** A proper exercise program should make getting a good night's sleep easier, not more difficult. If you're having more difficulty sleeping normally, decrease the amount of exercise you do until your symptoms subside.

✔ **Increased aches and pains in your joints:** Some muscle discomfort is inevitable when you start exercising after being very inactive. However, your joints should neither hurt nor continue feeling stiff. Make sure that you're warming up and stretching correctly. Muscle cramping and back discomfort also may indicate poor warm-up techniques. If symptoms persist, consult your physician.

Sounding medic alert: Symptoms to watch for during exercise

The key to safe exercise is never leaving your common sense at home. Staying in tune with any symptoms that you have during an exercise session is important for achieving maximum benefit and safety from exercising, especially when you're at risk for heart disease or already have established signs or symptoms or manifestations of heart disease. If the following symptoms occur during exercise, contact your physician before continuing your walking routine or any other form of physical activity.

✔ **Discomfort in the chest, arm, upper body, neck, or jaw:** These symptoms may very well be angina. If you have any questions, you need to discuss them with your doctor. This type of discomfort may be of any intensity and may be experienced as aching, burning, or a sensation of fullness or tightness.

✔ **Faintness or lightheadedness:** These symptoms may occur after exercise whenever your cool-down is too brief. This situation usually isn't serious and can be managed by extending the cool-down. However, if you experience a fainting spell or feel that you're about to faint during exercise, immediately discontinue the activity and consult your physician.

✔ **Excessive shortness of breath:** While you're walking or performing any other form of aerobic exercise, you can expect the rate and depth of your breathing to increase, but you shouldn't feel uncomfortable. A good rule to follow is that breathing should not be so difficult that talking becomes an effort. If wheezing develops or if recovery from shortness of breath takes more than five minutes at the conclusion of an exercise session, you need to consult with your doctor.

✔ **Irregular pulse:** If your pulse is irregular, skips, or races, either during or after exercise, such that it differs from your normal pulse, consulting your physician is important.

✔ **Changes in usual symptoms:** If your usual symptoms change — an increase in angina or shortness of breath, for example — or pain occurs or becomes more severe or persistent in an arthritic joint or at the site of a previous orthopedic injury, you need to consult with your physician.

✔ **Any other symptoms:** Finally, you always need to discuss any other symptoms that concern you with your physician. Exercise should be a pleasure and not a chore. Pain is a warning sign that you should never ignore.

Some medications can also affect the intensity of your exercise program but not its effectiveness. Discuss this possibility with your doctor.

How do medicines affect exercise?

People who already who have heart disease or risk factors for heart disease (such as hypertension or elevated blood cholesterol) often take medicines that may interact with exercise. Understanding which medicines may affect your exercise program is important.

✔ **Beta blockers:** Patients with heart disease and/or hypertension often are on a class of medicines known as beta blockers. These medicines lower blood pressure and thus decrease the work of the heart. They also keep your heart rate lower even when you exercise, which means that if you're taking a beta blocker, you need to gauge the intensity of your exercise by perceived exertion (see the earlier section "Easing on down the road — into a great start") rather than by heart rate. Remember to gauge your exercise to achieve moderate levels of exertion. People on beta blockers can achieve the same cardiac benefits from exercise as those who are not.

✔ **Calcium channel blockers:** Calcium channel blockers also are common medicines among patients who have heart disease or hypertension. Some of these medications also can lower the heart-rate response to exercise. Once again, the good news is that they don't prohibit you from achieving the multiple cardiac and other health benefits from regular physical activity.

✔ **Diuretics:** Diuretics are common medicines for patients who have high blood pressure or are experiencing heart failure. These meds won't reduce the benefit that physical activity provides for the heart; however, paying particular attention to adequate hydration when you're taking a diuretic is particularly important. Drink plenty of water before, during, and after physical activity. If you're on fluid restriction, consult your physician about fluid or water intake during exercise and be sure to monitor your weight daily.

Overcoming excuses

Everyone, even the most regular exerciser, faces periods when it is more difficult to exercise. Oftentimes, people who want to exercise are their own worst enemies because they make up excuses for not sticking with their exercise programs. Here are some common excuses and how to overcome them.

Excuse: I am busy. I don't have time.

Solution: Find a specific time to exercise and write it on your calendar or appointment book. Keep your appointment to exercise the same way you'd keep any other appointment.

Excuse: The weather is bad.

Solution: Always have a Plan B. Be ready for bad weather by finding a number of alternative locations for your walking program, such as a shopping mall or a fitness facility. Better yet, buy a treadmill and walk at home. Anticipate changes of season. For example, before the weather turns bitterly cold, be sure to plan where and when you're going to walk during the winter months.

Excuse: I am too tired.

Solution: You may be exercising too hard, if it makes you tired, but you may also want to consider exercising earlier in the day. Your walk should invigorate you. If it doesn't, you need to adjust your schedule or the intensity of your walk.

Excuse: Walking is boring! I don't look forward to it or enjoy it.

Solution: Vary your walking route. Employ different strategies, such as walking with family and friends. Join a group, such as the local mall-walking group, or walk while listening to a radio or tape player.

Excuse: Walking cuts into family time.

Solution: Ask your family members to join in your walking program. That way it benefits everyone!

Chapter 22

Reducing Stress: Tapping the Mind/Body Connection to Improve Heart Health

*T*he mind, the emotions, and the heart long have been linked in the human imagination. Since prehistoric times, people have identified the heart as the seat of love and other emotions.

- ✔ You give your heart to the ones you love.

- ✔ And when your heart breaks, you suffer *heartache,* which the dictionary defines as "anguish of mind."

- ✔ Like medieval knights swearing allegiance to their king, people still place hands over their physical hearts to pledge loyalty to their nations.

- ✔ A close call "makes your heart stop" and "scares you to death."

- ✔ If you fight bravely to the end in any cause, you "never lose heart," but if you give up easily, you're "fainthearted."

- ✔ Anger makes your "blood boil," but a positive, cheerful outlook makes you "lighthearted."

Humankind's prehistoric ancestors undoubtedly used the same telling expressions linking the mind and heart as they told stories around the fire in the family cave or confronted the woolly mammoth outside in the wilderness.

Even though modern science has taken a long time to begin to catch up with folklore and language, scientists are beginning to understand that powerful links between mind and body actually exist. Although emotional states and psychological health appear to have an impact on virtually every organ system, the links between the mind and heart probably have been the most fully studied and understood. In this chapter, I review links between stress, anger, love, friendship, intimacy, fear, and many other physiological states and cardiac health. I also review some simple strategies for controlling stress and anger and opening up your heart to promote cardiac health.

Understanding the Connections between Stress and the Heart

High stress levels constitute one of the cardiac health risks (and general health risks) that everyone faces daily. In fact, a growing body of scientific and medical evidence links stress to a variety of illnesses ranging from heart disease and cancer to the common cold. Unfortunately, stress is pervasive in today's modern, fast-paced society. One study from the National Institute of Mental Health found that more than 30 percent of adults experience enough stress in their daily lives to impair their performance at work or at home.

Defining stress

Despite literally hundreds of studies about stress, a precise definition is frustratingly difficult to come up with. Perhaps the best simple definition came from Canadian scientist Hans Selye, who in 1956 defined stress as "the nonspecific response of the body to any demands made on it" in his pioneering book *The Stress of Life*. The *demand* (the thing that stresses you out, be it a traffic jam, power outage, or deadline) and the *response* (your internal reaction to, say, a $1,500 car-repair bill or any other demand) are the key components of stress. No doubt you're faced with many demands (stressors) every day. How you respond is up to you, but remember that the way you respond can contribute either to improved cardiac health or to increased cardiac risk.

Describing positive versus negative stress

Many people don't realize that having positive stress is possible. But a certain amount of stress may be necessary for you to reach your optimal performance. For example, outstanding athletes often perform at their best in the "big game." And you may be one of the many people who work best when faced with a deadline. However, when stress becomes excessive or when your response to the stress becomes negative, your health in general, and your cardiac health in particular, may be harmed.

Linking stress to heart disease

When it comes to the heart, stress can

- ✔ Increase your likelihood of developing coronary artery disease (CAD)
- ✔ Create chest discomfort that can mimic heart disease
- ✔ Cause palpitations or even very serious arrhythmias
- ✔ Contribute to the development of high blood pressure

Numerous scientific studies link job-related stress to an increase in the likelihood of your developing coronary artery disease. Some of these studies show that heart attacks occur more often during the six months following negative life changes, such as divorce, financial setback, or the death of a spouse or close relative than they do during the six months before these negative life changes. Although this evidence isn't as strong as the evidence that links heart disease to other established major risk factors, such as elevated cholesterol, cigarette smoking, and physical inactivity, it nevertheless is strong enough to make stress a risk factor for heart disease (see Chapter 3).

Linking stress to high blood pressure

The link between stress and high blood pressure is well established. Many years ago, Dr. Walter Cannon, a famous physiologist, coined the phrase *fight or flight* to describe the physiological changes that occur during stress. He linked this response to the genetic makeup of humans. When confronted by a dangerous and frightening saber-toothed tiger, for example, ancient human ancestors needed to make an immediate decision whether to stand and fight, freeze with fear, or immediately take flight. One physiological response to this stress is elevated blood pressure.

Unfortunately, people still have the genetic makeup that causes their blood pressure to rise during emotionally stressful situations. For example, studies show that air-traffic controllers, whose jobs place them under continually high levels of stress, are more likely to have high blood pressure than people in many other professions.

Constant pressure caused by events and situations over which you feel you have only minimal control is a particularly dangerous form of stress. For example, blood pressure rises in soldiers during times of war, in civilians faced with natural disasters, such as floods or explosions, and in entire societies in which social order is unstable.

Linking Type A personality traits to heart problems

About 40 years ago, Dr. Ray Rosenman and Dr. Meyer Friedman developed the concept of *Type A Personality,* which links certain kinds of behavior and personality traits with an increased incidence of heart attack. Unfortunately, the concept of Type A behavior often is loosely and incorrectly applied to any hard-driving, busy worker.

The research defines Type A behavior, however, as containing aggression, competitiveness, and hostility. Individuals who exhibit true Type A behavior also are likely to have a sense of incredible urgency as they attempt to accomplish poorly defined goals in the shortest period of time. Likewise, they often are angry when confronted with unexpected delays. The combination of *frustration* and *anger* is essential to manifest the cardiac danger associated with a Type A personality. Hard workers who are happy in their work, even when they're workaholics, are more likely to fall into what Rosenman and Friedman characterized as *Type B personalities* and are not at increased risk of heart disease.

Linking anger to dangerous heart problems

Recent studies from a variety of investigators, including Dr. Redford Williams at Duke University, show that the hostility component of Type A behavior specifically accounts for almost all the increased risk of cardiac disease. Using one of the subscales on psychological inventories administered to many participants in large heart-health trials, Dr. Williams and his colleagues identified cynical mistrust of others, frequent experience of angry feelings, and overt expression of cynicism and anger in aggressive behavior as key factors that make up the psychological profile that increases the risk of developing heart disease. In real-life situations, this discovery points not only to the knowledge that anger kills when you let it control your behavior — think road rage — but also to the knowledge that it may also kill by damaging your heart.

Making Connections: Friendship, Intimacy, and Cardiac Health

People who have trouble connecting with others and developing intimate relationships also may have a higher risk of developing heart disease and suffering its consequences. The opposite also is true: Those who have strong relationships with others also have a healthier heart.

Suffering the lonely heart

Maybe poets are absolutely correct when they write about dying of a broken heart. Numerous studies show that individuals who feel isolated and alone are much more likely to experience health problems, including heart disease and cancer, than are individuals who experience intimacy, love, and a sense of being connected. Take a look at the findings:

✔ The prestigious *New England Journal of Medicine* published a study of more than 2,300 men who had survived a heart attack, The risk of death for participants who were classified as socially isolated and having a high degree of stress was more than four times that of participants with low levels of stress and isolation. These relationships held up even when the study was controlled for other cardiac risk factors, such as smoking, diet, exercise, and weight.

✔ In a Duke University study of 1,400 men and women who had blockage of at least one coronary artery (determined by coronary angiography), study participants who weren't married and didn't have at least one close confidant were more than three times more likely to have died at follow-up than participants who were married and/or had a confidant.

✔ In a third study, participants who suffered a recent heart attack and lived alone experienced twice the risk of dying after a heart attack when compared with participants who lived with one or more other individuals and described their relationships as close.

In many other studies conducted in diverse cultures, social isolation has been found to increase the risk of heart disease, sudden death, and cancer.

Promoting the healing power of love

Numerous studies show that people who give and receive love actually decrease their risks of heart disease and other diseases. Check out these examples:

✔ In one famous study conducted among Harvard undergraduates in the early 1950s, participants were asked to describe their relationships with their parents. When their medical records were examined in the 1980s, the results were astounding. Ninety-one percent of these former students who said they didn't have a loving relationship with their parents had been diagnosed with serious diseases by midlife, most prominently CAD and high blood pressure. However, fewer than 50 percent of the participants who reported warm and loving relationships with their parents had developed these chronic diseases in adult life.

✔ A similar study conducted at Johns Hopkins Medical School shows that physician participants who ultimately developed severe medical

problems were much less likely to have described close loving relationships earlier in life than were participants who had not suffered such
medical problems.

✔ In yet another study of elderly individuals with heart disease, participants who were able to reach out for help had one-third the risk of dying
from heart disease as older individuals who tried to go it alone.

Connecting for heart health

As you can see, the ability to connect with other individuals appears to carry
significant cardiac benefit. If you feel isolated or lonely, it may be time to
make some connections by

✔ Investing time and thought in friends and/or family as seriously as you
do in your work.

✔ Joining an interest group. From chess clubs to gardening clubs, book
clubs to folkdance societies, running clubs to writing classes, an activity-
related group that matches your interests is out there for you to benefit
from.

✔ Finding a third place. Beyond home and work, people long have bene-
fited from a close connection to a *third place* in their communities. For
many it's their church, synagogue, mosque, or temple. For others, it's a
social group, community organization, or other activity or group that is
meaningful to them. The identity of your third place isn't as important as
the fact that you have one.

Being "Scared to Death" and Other Mind/Body Links

Everybody has experienced a racing heart — after a bad scare or an angry
moment, for instance. Strong emotion also can produce serious rhythm
disturbances (see Chapter 6).

Understanding that mind/body links are hardwired

Although feelings of joy, anger, or depression may be complex functions, your
body has only a limited vocabulary of physiological responses to them. Most
of these responses are mediated through the nervous system, which controls
all your body's functions.

The nervous system is divided into two major branches: the *sympathetic nervous system* and the *parasympathetic nervous system.*

✔ When the sympathetic nervous system (the part of the nervous system that results in the fight or flight response) is stimulated, various rhythm disturbances caused by rapid heartbeat or extra beats can occur. Fear and anger are two stimuli that trigger this system. Stress can also cause palpitations that typically are experienced by individuals as skipped heartbeats or irregular heartbeats.

✔ When the parasympathetic nervous system (the part of the nervous system that is responsible for maintenance of routine body function, also called *rest and digest functions*) is stimulated, a slow heart rate can result. The most common result of an excessively slow heartbeat is fainting. Typically any condition that produces a faint — crowded room, hot day, having blood drawn — triggers this system.

People who are more susceptible to rhythm abnormalities provoked by emotion also are more likely to have underlying cardiac disease, particularly CAD. But occasionally people with normal coronary arteries develop severe cardiac arrhythmias in stressful settings.

"Dropping dead" from stress — myth or reality?

Plenty of anecdotal evidence points to the fact that people may collapse and die when faced with sudden overwhelming emotional stress. Dr. George Engel, a leading researcher in this area, reviewed a number of cases in which psychological stress appeared to cause sudden death. He found that sudden death commonly took place during one of the following events:

✔ Hearing of the death of a friend or relative

✔ Suffering an acute episode of grief

✔ Mourning a sad event or its anniversary

✔ Losing status or self-esteem

✔ Experiencing personal threat or danger

✔ Experiencing a reunion or triumph

Specific evidence often is lacking in these situations, but experts believe that in most of these circumstances the sudden death results from a severe form of cardiac arrhythmia called *ventricular tachycardia,* which ultimately degenerates into a fatal cardiac arrhythmia called *ventricular fibrillation,* where the heart ineffectively quivers and is unable to pump out blood. (See Chapter 6.)

Understanding stress caused by heart problems

In much the same way that psychological stress can result in either acute or chronic heart problems, the flip side is also true — heart disease can result in psychological problems.

The period *after* a heart attack (see also Chapter 5) has drawn the most attention from researchers. Many people go through a three-part psychological response to having a heart attack that includes

✔ Initially experiencing great anxiety produced by the physical event of heart attack and by fear of dying.

✔ Denying that you've had a heart attack or denying that anything is seriously wrong with you.

✔ Settling into what is known as *homecoming depression.* In this situation, you may become depressed and worried about the long-term consequences of your heart attack or become remorseful about lifestyle practices that may have contributed to your cardiac problem.

During and after a heart attack, psychological stress typically diminishes when the patient is surrounded by caring, supportive health-care workers and family. Studies show that individuals who have such strong support systems are much more likely to recover from a heart attack than individuals who do not.

Understanding the heart attack that isn't: Heart disease mimics

Studies show that 10 percent to 20 percent of cardiac patients may have symptoms caused not by their heart disease but instead by underlying emotional disorders. Perhaps an equal number of individuals who don't have heart disease visit their physicians with manifestations of underlying emotional problems that may initially be confused with heart disease. The three most common emotional disorders that can mimic heart disease are

✔ **Anxiety states:** The spectrum of anxiety states extends from chronic anxiety through attacks of anxiety in specific settings. Such anxiety states often may be accompanied by rapid heartbeat, palpitations, chest pain, or tightness or shortness of breath. Although these symptoms need to be taken seriously, a physician typically can rule out serious cardiac disease. Anxiety states typically respond well to support and reassurance, including psychological counseling and therapy whenever necessary.

✔ **Panic disorder:** Although panic disorder is one of the anxiety states, its presentation may be so dramatic and so similar to cardiovascular disease that it deserves separate consideration. Individuals with panic disorder can experience a sudden outpouring of feelings of terror and impending doom. These may be accompanied by chest pain, severe shortness of breath, and irregular heartbeat — symptoms that may resemble serious cardiac disease. Attacks often occur in predictable settings, such as crowded rooms, theaters, or other public places where exit may be restricted. A physician typically can distinguish between a panic disorder and serious heart disease. Taking a careful history is important to making the right diagnosis.

✔ **Depression:** Considerable overlap exists between depression and heart disease. Sometimes people who have heart disease become depressed, and in other instances, medicines used to treat high blood pressure or CAD tend to have side effects that may cause depression. Treatment of the underlying depression typically resolves all symptoms in such cases.

Understanding how psychotropic medications may affect the heart

Psychotropic medications act on the mind (*psyche* = mind; *tropic* = influencing) and often are prescribed for anxiety or for depression. Psychotropic medications have made it easier to manage these conditions effectively, and they are prescribed for large numbers of people. However, many medications that work on the brain may also affect the heart. For example, some medicines used for treating depression may contribute to rapid heartbeat and palpitations.

If you suffer from depression, taking your medication is important, and most antidepressant medications are safe. But if you also have heart disease, you may want to discuss with your doctor any potential side effects taking any of these medicines may have on the heart.

Keeping Stress and Anger at Bay

Do you get bent out of shape when the weather ruins your plans? When a driver cuts you off? When a last-minute project keeps you late at work? If you do, you're risking serious damage to your heart, which can stand up to only so much stress and anger. Reducing these risk factors is up to you, and it's not as hard as you may think.

Controlling stress with a four-part plan

Stress may be dangerous for the heart, but the good news is that some simple strategies may significantly lower stress and thereby improve cardiac health. Here are four ways to lower the stress in your life and contribute to cardiac health:

✔ **Modify or eliminate circumstances that contribute to stress and cardiac symptoms.**

People often simply do not realize that aspects of their daily lives can compound problems with stress. Cutting back on caffeinated beverages, such as coffee, tea, and many soft drinks, for example, may make a substantial difference in your stress levels and manifestations like cardiac palpitations. Fatigue and insomnia may also contribute to stress, so be sure that you get plenty of rest and a good night's sleep whenever you're experiencing symptoms of stress. You also need to avoid the temptation to use alcohol as a way to relax. Although it may seem to offer a temporary release from stress, it usually leads to greater problems.

✔ **Live in the present.**

The basis for all effective stress reduction is being able to live in the present. It may sound simple, but many people spend an inordinate amount of time either regretting the past or fearing the future. Strategies such as biofeedback, visualization, and medications can help you live in the present and substantially lower stress levels.

✔ **Get out of your own way.**

Many people compound the inevitable stresses of their daily lives by layering on negative feelings concerning these stresses. Recognizing that no one can live a life that is completely free of stress is as important as trying not to compound the problem by allowing feelings of negativity or low self-worth to make stress worse.

✔ **Develop a personal plan for stress.**

Developing a personal plan to alleviate stress is one of the most effective ways to handle it on an ongoing basis, instead of allowing it to become free-floating anxiety. Many people find that daily exercise, meditation, taking a timeout (either alone or with family), and other such strategies provide effective ways of controlling the stresses of daily life.

Ten-minute timeouts against stress

"Step away for ten a day": Short, calming breaks from your daily routine can lower your stress dramatically. Try one of these techniques:

Go outside. The right short break outside can ease the tension.

Do: Stroll. Clear your mind. Smell the flowers. People watch.

Don't: Think about your schedule. Outline that memo. Pick at a worry.

Tune into calm. You can also get away right in your office or easy chair. Simply find a quiet, comfortable spot. Allow no interruptions. Sit quietly and focus on becoming calm. Consciously clear your mind, gently pushing away any intruding thoughts of work or problems. Listening to quiet music, visualizing peaceful scenes, or focusing on deep, slow breathing may help. A luxurious stretch at the end of your ten minutes can be a nice transition back to activity.

Listen to your body. Using biofeedback techniques can help you foster a relaxed state. In research conducted in my laboratory, I found that people who take ten minutes each day to focus on relaxing were able to dramatically reduce their stress levels. They used the same techniques that I described earlier, but they also relied on a heart-rate monitor as their point of focus. Sitting quietly, focus on your heart rate and imagine it going lower. Using the other visualization techniques in combination with biofeedback can enhance your ten-minute timeout.

Meditate. Practicing any of several formal types of meditation can be useful to anyone who enjoys it. *Meditation For Dummies* (Wiley) can get you started.

Catnap. If you're one of those lucky souls who can drop instantly to sleep and wake refreshed in 10 or 15 minutes, you can experience the ten-minute timeout in one of its most satisfying forms (at least, so say its devotees).

Controlling anger with five simple steps

The hostility or anger component of the Type A personality poses the most significant cardiac risk. Here are five simple strategies for helping you control anger:

✔ **Learn how to trust other people.** An open heart is a healthy heart. Individuals who are isolated and fearful of other people increase their risk of cardiac disease. By making an effort to open yourself up to trusting other individuals, you can substantially lower your risk of heart disease.

✔ **Plant a garden and care for a pet.** The Irish poet William Butler Yeats said the definition of a civilized human being is one who plants a garden and cares for a domestic pet. This concept is not only a prescription for a civilized human being, but also a prescription for a heart-healthy life.

✔ **Practice asserting yourself.** Many people keep their emotions bottled up inside. They're often pleasantly surprised to find out that by standing up for what they believe (in a pleasant way, of course), they can control unwarranted stress in their lives and lead a happier daily existence.

✔ **Become a volunteer.** A wonderful body of literature suggests that volunteers not only do good for other people, but they also improve their own health. Somehow, the act of giving of yourself to other people results in improved health for yourself.

✔ **Practice forgiveness.** Many people keep themselves in a constant state of anger for wrongs or supposed slights from other people or from the world at large. Learning how to forgive others is one of the very best things that you can do to improve your own cardiac health. While you're at it, forgive yourself, too, for past shortcomings — imagined or real.

Chapter 23

Quitting Smoking

. . . .

. . . .

*O*nly one good thing can be said about cigarette smoking — it's good when you stop! In the United States, cigarette smoking is responsible for an enormous amount of unnecessary suffering and death every year.

✔ Cigarette smoking is the leading cause of preventable death in the U.S., claiming more than 400,000 lives per year.

✔ Depending on the amount of cigarette smoking you do, it increases your risk of heart disease between 200 percent and 400 percent.

✔ Smoking increases your risk of lung cancer by 20 to 30 times.

✔ Smoking harms the people around you through secondhand smoke, which can lead to angina attacks in people with coronary artery disease (CAD) and may result in chronic bronchitis in children who live with smokers.

But guess what? None of this information is news to people who smoke cigarettes. As a friend of mine once said, "Everyone who doesn't exercise knows that they should, and everyone who smokes cigarettes knows that they shouldn't!"

So I'm not going to rattle off too many statistics about why you need to stop smoking. Instead, I'll simply review enough about how smoking relates to coronary heart disease to give your willpower extra ammunition against the urges of your nicotine habit or to reinforce your commitment to supporting someone who's trying to quit. After that, I discuss some specific recommendations for *how to* stop smoking. For the good of your heart and overall health, it's never too late to quit.

Affirming Reasons for Not Smoking

Cigarette smoke harms virtually every vital organ, but it is particularly dangerous to the heart and lungs. Incidentally, anyone who thinks they're safe using smokeless tobacco, cigars, or pipes needs to think again. More about going smokeless in the section "Reviewing the Dangers of Other Forms of Tobacco" later in the chapter.

Linking cigarette smoking and heart disease

As a cardiologist, I'm astounded that so many people still don't appreciate just how serious the link is between cigarette smoking and heart disease.

Depending on how much they smoke, cigarette smokers increase their risk of developing heart disease two to four times more than nonsmokers. In fact, every cigarette that you light up increases your blood pressure, and the nicotine you take in causes coronary arteries to mildly constrict. This problem is bad enough in a normal person, but for someone who suffers with angina, it can bring on significant symptoms.

Cigarette smoking also increases the bad cholesterol (LDL) and decreases the good cholesterol (HDL) in your bloodstream. Smoking also significantly increases your risk of developing peripheral vascular disease and aortic disease.

Linking cigarette smoking with other diseases

Smoking accounts for 25 percent of all cancer deaths in the U.S., including 87 percent of lung cancer deaths. Smoking also is associated with cancers of the mouth and throat (all structures), esophagus (food tube), pancreas, cervix, kidney, and bladder. Want more bad news? Cigarette smoking is associated with such annoying, chronic conditions as the common cold, stomach ulcers, chronic bronchitis and many other lung diseases, and with catastrophic events, such as stroke.

Considering smoking and women

For reasons that aren't completely clear, cigarette smoking appears to be particularly dangerous for women. In fact, some studies suggest that the risk of heart attack in women who smoke is approximately 50 percent greater than the risk in male smokers. One possible explanation for this increased risk for women is the interaction between the chemicals in cigarette smoke and female hormones. In addition, lung cancer is now the leading cause of cancer death in women in the U.S., having surpassed breast cancer in 1987.

Considering smoking and children

More than 90 percent of current smokers started when they were children. Sadly, every day an estimated 4,800 children younger than 18 smoke their first cigarettes, and 2,000 of these youngsters will become regular smokers. More than 71 percent of high school students have tried cigarette smoking, and 28 percent of high school students currently smoke cigarettes.

If you never start smoking as a child, however, you're unlikely ever to start smoking. If you're a young smoker, the best thing you can do for your long-term good health is kick the tobacco habit now.

Considering smoking and African Americans

Cigarette smoking also appears particularly dangerous for African Americans, who have higher levels of the nicotine and its byproducts in their blood than Caucasian smokers. And for reasons that aren't completely clear, African Americans who smoke appear more susceptible to heart disease than Caucasians. In addition, African Americans are at greater risk of high blood pressure, which also is negatively affected by smoking.

Considering the dangers of secondhand smoke

People who live or work with active cigarette smokers are susceptible to *secondhand smoke* (also called passive smoke, environmental tobacco smoke, or ETS), which enters the air from lighted cigarettes or the exhalations of smokers. Every year, 35,000 to 45,000 deaths from heart disease and 3,000 deaths from cancer are attributed to secondhand smoke. Secondhand smoke also is responsible for between 150,000 and 300,000 respiratory tract infections annually.

Checking out the benefits of quitting

Before you get too depressed about all the bad news associated with ciga-rette smoking, take a look at the bright side:

✔ Every year, about 1.2 million smokers are able to quit successfully. After only one year of not smoking, the excess cardiac risk from smoking is cut in half. Fifteen years after you stop smoking, your risk is similar to that of a person who never smoked.

✔ Male smokers who quit between the ages of 35 and 40 add an average of five years to their lives. Female smokers who quit at the same time add three years to their lives. And it's never too late to quit. Even men and women who quit between the ages of 65 and 69 can increase their life expectancies. In one recent study, 65-year-old women who quit smoking added an average of four years to their life expectancies.

✔ Quitting smoking is truly possible. With modern smoking cessation pro-grams, 20 percent to 40 percent of participants successfully stop smok-ing. New aids now in the marketplace that help people quit smoking may help this success rate climb even higher.

Understanding Nicotine Addiction: A Chain That Binds

Nicotine is a powerfully addictive drug. Using nicotine causes changes in the brain that compel people to use it more and more. In addition, attempting to stop using nicotine causes unpleasant physical and emotional side effects. Good feelings when the drug is present combined with bad feelings when the drug is not present are the hallmarks of addiction. And many researchers judge nicotine to be as addicting as heroin and cocaine.

Examining what nicotine does to the body

When you smoke a cigarette, ingesting the chemical nicotine causes a number of immediate responses in your body. In the short term, your blood pressure and heart rate rise, and the arteries supplying your heart narrow. When these arteries narrow, the combination of nicotine and carbon monox-ide spell double trouble to your heart, because carbon monoxide reduces the amount of oxygen that the blood can carry. In addition, smoking causes abnormalities in the way that your body handles various fats (causing a rise in the bad cholesterol LDL and a decrease in the good cholesterol HDL) and affects various hormones and how the body handles blood sugar.

Understanding nicotine's impact on the heart

Cigarette smoking harms the heart and the arteries. Carbon monoxide in cigarette smoke appears to damage the walls of arteries and encourages the buildup of fat along these walls. Nicotine may also contribute to this process. In addition, chemicals in cigarette smoke make blood platelets stickier and thereby increase the likelihood that your blood will clot. All these effects combined significantly increase the risk of heart disease.

Checking out nicotine replacement products

Many smokers who want to quit turn to *nicotine replacement products* such as nicotine transdermal patches, nicotine gum, and nicotine inhalers. These products have been successful in helping smokers quit when they're used as part of an overall comprehensive program to quit smoking. Nicotine, of course, is still nicotine, and it's still addictive. But nicotine replacement is different from smoking in at least two important physical ways. First, when using nicotine replacements, you avoid inhaling harmful carbon monoxide, tars, and other toxins that are present in smoke. Second, when you smoke, nicotine is delivered to your brain in a sudden rush that tapers off over a couple of hours. Nicotine replacements deliver nicotine to your body at a steadier rate without your having to *take a hit* from a cigarette.

Getting away from that hit of nicotine may make quitting easier. At any rate, such nicotine substitutions appear to help ease some of the psychological and physiological problems associated with withdrawal from nicotine. In an optimal situation, you should work with your doctor when using nicotine replacement therapy, even though nicotine patches and gum now are available over the counter.

If you're diagnosed with any form of heart disease, never use any nicotine replacement product without discussing it with your physician. In general, unsupervised nicotine-replacement therapy is not recommended for patients with heart or circulatory problems.

Reviewing the Dangers of Other Forms of Tobacco

Although this chapter focuses mainly on cigarette smoking, no form of tobacco is safe. Here's a look at some of the other forms of tobacco use:

- ✔ **Smokeless tobacco:** The use of all forms of smokeless tobacco, including plug, leaf, and snuff, is on the rise, according to recent data. Such products often are referred to as *spit tobacco.* Perhaps the greatest cause for concern is the highly addictive practice of *dipping snuff,* which is when tobacco (either moist leaf snuff or dry powdered snuff) is placed between the cheek and the gum. Nicotine and other cancer-causing agents are absorbed through the gum tissues and expose the body to levels of nicotine equal to those of cigarette smoking. The nicotine from smokeless tobacco poses dangers similar to those from cigarettes. In addition, individuals who dip snuff have a greatly increased risk of developing mouth and throat cancers, which are among the most difficult to treat effectively.

- ✔ **Cigars:** What price glitter and phony sophistication? During the last decade, cigar consumption has doubled. And although the sale of expensive cigars isn't growing as fast as it was during the 1990s, sales of all cigars remain steady. Regardless of the elitist, stylish image hyped in slick magazines, cigar smoking is extremely hazardous to your health. Almost all the same cancer-causing agents found in cigarettes also are found in cigars. But the overall death rate is increased by almost 40 percent in individuals who smoke cigars when compared with nonsmokers. The increased risk of mouth cancers is between 500 percent and 1,000 percent. Oh, so you don't inhale the smoke? Well then, exactly what is that blue haze hanging about that trendy bar or in your living room?

- ✔ **Pipe smoking:** Although less data is available about smoking pipes than cigars, there is no reason to doubt that pipes are just as dangerous as cigars. Pipe smokers certainly experience increased cancers of the lip and mouth.

Taking Steps to Stop Smoking

One of the first things you need to do when you decide to quit smoking is set up a firm foundation for a successful campaign by considering the following guidelines. These tips are based on reviews of plenty of research, and they're consistent with the recommendations for quitting from a number of health agencies.

✔ **Be committed.** Breaking the nicotine addiction isn't easy. It takes an enormous individual effort. But you can be encouraged by the fact that half the people who ever smoked cigarettes have quit.

✔ **Talk to your doctor.** Ask your physician about nicotine replacement therapy and other available programs to help you quit smoking. This type of communication helps maximize your chances of success.

✔ **Set a quit date.** Studies show that you're more likely to stop smoking if you set a specific date instead of trying to taper off.

✔ **Build on past mistakes.** The average cigarette smoker usually tries to quit smoking six to ten times before doing so successfully. Review what has worked and what has not worked for you during past efforts.

✔ **Seek the support of family and friends.** Tell your family and friends that you're trying to quit smoking and enlist them in your efforts to stop. If they're truly your friends, they'll be supportive.

✔ **Learn how to cope.** Most cigarette smoking is triggered by other cues. Try minimizing or working around the cues in your life that stimulate you to smoke.

✔ **Take the focus off weight gain.** True, many people who stop smoking gain some weight, but the vast majority of them gain fewer than ten pounds. The health benefits of quitting smoking far outweigh the risks of the small weight gain that some people experience when they stop.

✔ **Avoid dieting while trying to stop smoking.** Remember that famous slogan for success: KISS! (Keep it simple, stupid!) Trying to change too many things at once is an invitation for failure.

If these guidelines aren't enough, you may want to give *Quitting Smoking For Dummies* (Wiley) by Dr. David Brizer a try. It can provide you with what you need to know to quit.

Using Helpful Aids to Stop Smoking

A number of different options are available to help you stop smoking. Recent research shows that three particular program elements are particularly effective when used either alone or together to help smokers quit.

✔ **Nicotine replacement therapy:** Using these nicotine replacement products, such as nicotine patches, gum, inhalers, and nasal spray, increases the likelihood of quitting successfully. Nicotine patches and gum can now be obtained without a prescription. Nicotine nasal sprays and inhalers also have been approved by the Food and Drug Administration (FDA) and may be helpful for some individuals. Talk to your doctor about some of the prescription medications that now are available.

✔ **Social support:** Receiving encouragement and support from your physician and your family is important. Support from others who are trying to quit smoking may also be helpful. Various smoking cessation groups are sure to be meeting in your area (community-based and commercial). And you may even want to try an online support group like the one that QuitNet (`www.quitnet.org`) provides. For other online groups and resources type in `smoking cessation` as the search term on your Web browser. Although that term sounds a bit stiff and technical, you'll probably get the best results with it. I also provide additional resources at the end of this chapter.

✔ **Skills training/problem-solving:** Listening to the practical advice and techniques that physicians, other health-care workers, smoking-cessation specialists, and people who've quit can provide is extremely helpful when you're trying to quit smoking. More than 30 states now have telephone *quit lines* you can call to speak with a counselor about your plan and available resources.

Group and individual counseling also can help. Counseling needs to be intensive and last for at least two weeks but preferably up to eight weeks.

Other techniques that may help you quit smoking include acupuncture and hypnosis. In all instances, these aids should be used in conjunction with an overall comprehensive program prescribed by your physician and/or smoking cessation specialist.

Developing a Specific Plan to Quit

A variety of sources offer excellent information to help smokers break the habit. Some particularly helpful resources were developed by the National Cancer Institute (NCI — your tax dollars at work in a good cause). You can review these resources online at `cancer.gov` and `smokefree.gov`, or you can ask for printed resources that are free-of-charge from the NCI by calling 800-422-6237.

Here are key recommendations adapted from the National Cancer Institute materials:

✔ **Prepare yourself to quit.** After you decide to quit, list all the reasons why you want to quit, and get yourself ready. Set a target date for quitting, perhaps a special day such as a birthday, or anniversary, or the Great American Smokeout, which takes place annually on the third Thursday in November.

✔ **Know what to expect.** Be realistic. You're going to experience some withdrawal symptoms, but they usually last only one to two weeks.

✔ **Involve someone else.** Get the support of your family, friends, and physician. Maybe even ask another smoker to quit with you. You can't overestimate the importance of support.

✔ **Before your quit day, you may want to prepare yourself with these techniques:**

- Switch brands. Find one that you find distasteful.

- Cut down the number of cigarettes that you smoke each day.

- Try not to smoke automatically (after meals and phone calls, for example).

- Make smoking inconvenient. Go outside to smoke when it's cold or raining, go to malls or movies where smoking is prohibited, and so on.

- Clean your clothes to get rid of the smell of cigarettes.

✔ **On the day that you quit, use these strategies:**

- Throw away all your cigarettes, matches, and lighters; if you can't stand to throw away your collection of ashtrays, store them in the most inaccessible corner of your attic.

- Keep busy with plenty of activities on the big quit day. Remind your family and friends, so they can be extrasupportive.

- Think about things that you'd like to buy for yourself. Estimate their cost in terms of packs of cigarettes and put aside the money to buy these presents.

- At the end of the day, buy yourself a treat or celebrate.

✔ **Immediately after you quit, adopt these techniques:**

- Develop a clean, fresh nonsmoking environment. Buy flowers now that you can enjoy their scents.

- Drink large quantities of water.

- If you miss the sensation of having a cigarette in your hand, find something else to keep your hands and fingers occupied.

- Look for ways to minimize your temptation and to develop new habits, such as exercise. Exercising decreases yet another risk factor for heart disease.

- Don't worry about gaining a small amount of weight, but do make sure that you have a well-balanced diet. As the appetite-depressing effect of nicotine disappears, avoid replacing cigarettes with calorie-dense candy, cookies, and snack foods. Try sugarfree gum or fresh fruits instead. Doing so helps you deal with the common experience of gaining some weight after you stop smoking.

Relapsing is not collapsing

If you slip and start to smoke again, don't be discouraged or give up. Remember, most smokers have to try several times before they finally succeed at quitting. Don't be too hard on yourself, and get back on the nonsmoking track as quickly as possible.

Quitting for keeps

As you keep the faith — and fight the good fight — not smoking eventually becomes a part of you. You develop your own techniques and strategies for sustaining the positive feeling and pride that having stopped smoking gives you. Remaining vigilant about what triggers your smoking urge is important for a long time after you quit. When that old urge kicks in, make a mental note about what was going on when it happened. What were you doing? Where were you? Who were you with? What were you thinking? Check off the things that may trigger you to want to smoke and try counteracting them with specific strategies. Never give up — you can do it!

Finding More Information

Many different resources are available to help you in your fight to stop smoking. Here are a few organizations and Web sites:

- ✔ **The National Cancer Institute** provides great information at two Web sites and runs the Smokefree.gov project (www.smokefree.gov), where you can find a comprehensive guide to quitting, look up local and state quit line phone numbers, and talk to experts via e-mail. Phone: 800-422-6237; Web sites: www.nci.nih.gov and www.cancer.gov.

- ✔ **The American Cancer Society** offers the *Complete Guide to Quitting* free at its Web site (www.cancer.org). Phone: 800-227-2345.

- ✔ **Nicotine Anonymous** conducts a 12-step support program. Use its Web site (www.nicotine-anonymous.org) to locate meetings or find literature.

- ✔ **The American Heart Association** offers resources about why and how to quit, statistics about smoking, and articles about smoking's effects on your body. Phone: 800-242-8721; Web site: ww.americanheart.org.

- ✔ **The American Lung Association** has a popular quit-smoking course that's now available as a seven-module, interactive, online course. Look for "Freedom from Smoking Online" on the ALA homepage. Phone: 212-315-8700; Web site: www.lungusa.org.

Part VI
The Part of Tens

The 5th Wave By Rich Tennant

FITNESS SCHED.
MONDAY

SKIP ROPE
WEIGHTS
CRUNCHES
SQUATS

"I _AM_ following the schedule! Today I skipped the rope, then I skipped the weights, then I skipped the crunches..."

In this part . . .

Find the facts that bust the most common myths about heart disease. Check out which heart-healthy foods you can use to fine-tune your nutrition plan. I also show you when to take symptoms that signal heart disease to the doctor. I round out this section with ten secrets for long-term success in heart-healthy living.

Chapter 24

Ten Myths about Heart Disease

In This Chapter
▶ Busting myths before they bust your heart
▶ Avoiding misconceptions that lead to unwise choices

*I*t's no surprise that myths about heart disease often prevail. After all, the heart is a truly mythic organ — the fount of all life. Throughout the world's cultures, heroes and heroines of mythology and legend usually are persons of great heart. The same can be said of persons of great cunning. Their hearts are the embodiment of the courageous lifestyles that inspire the masses. But although myths can and do inspire, they also can kill . . . particularly the many myths surrounding heart disease. So let's bust a few.

The Myth of Modern Maturity

Heart disease is a disease of middle age and older years.

Many people think of heart disease as a problem of middle and older age, because that's when the manifestations of heart disease, such as angina and heart attack, strike. What a dangerous myth. Although the *manifestations* of coronary artery disease typically occur during the middle and later years of life, the *roots* of coronary artery disease lie in childhood. Using the heart-healthy lifestyle measures recommended in this book not only will help you but also will enable you to set an example for your children and grandchildren.

The Myth of the Old-Boy Network

Men are much more likely to get heart disease than women.

Way too many women think that heart disease is mainly a male disease. However, heart disease is by far the leading cause of death for women. Women are six to ten times more likely to die of heart disease than breast cancer (which women fear more). When cardiovascular disease and stroke are combined, these two diseases claim more female lives every year than the next 16 causes of death combined. Even so, many of these deaths are preventable. Using the daily lifestyle measures I present in this book can stop this equal-opportunity killer.

The Myth of Thomas Wolfe

Once you have heart disease, it is relentlessly progressive.

If you've been reading this book cover to cover, you know that Thomas Wolfe wrote the novel, *You Can't Go Home Again*. Until the last 15 years, coronary artery disease appeared to be a relentless lifelong process that resulted in increasing symptoms and, ultimately, death. Fortunately, during the last decade, doctors have found that following a low-fat, heart-healthy diet and a regimen of physical activity, usually in conjunction with taking cholesterol-lowering medications, can often halt the process of atherosclerosis (clogging of the arteries) in its tracks and sometimes even reverse the process to some degree. See Chapter 19 for details about how to turn down the path toward heading home to healthier, more normal arteries.

The Eisenhower Myth

After you've had a heart attack, your life will move inexorably downhill.

In 1954, President Dwight Eisenhower suffered a heart attack while in office — a first. His cardiologist, Dr. Paul Dudley White, from Harvard Medical School and Massachusetts General Hospital, appeared on national television to assure the anxious public that if President Eisenhower paid attention to what he ate and became involved in a regular walking program, he could continue to fulfill the strenuous duties of the highest office in the land. Most people were surprised to hear it. As Ike proved, you have no reason whatsoever to give up after you've had a heart attack. Modern cardiac rehabilitation can help people who've suffered a heart attack or have other serious forms of heart disease to live full, vigorous lives for many years after they experience the first manifestations of heart disease. See Chapter 18 for more details about modern cardiac rehabilitation.

The Myth of No Pain, No Gain

To get cardiac benefit from exercise, you need to get sweaty and out of breath.

Many sedentary individuals (and, indeed, many exercisers!) share the myth that you have to exercise at a fairly intense level to achieve cardiac benefits. To some degree, this myth grew from the advice of well-intentioned exercise physiologists, who said that improving your aerobic fitness requires at least three or four 20- to 30-minute sessions of continuous vigorous exercise every week. Without question, this advice is excellent if your only goal is improving your aerobic capacity. However, if your goal is lowering your risk of heart disease, totally different rules apply . . . you simply need to become more active. By more active, I mean trying to *accumulate* 30 minutes of *moderate* physical activity on most, if not all, days. Don't let the myth that you have to sweat like crazy for 30 minutes straight keep you and your heart declining . . . uh, reclining on the couch. See Chapter 21 to find out how to get started.

The Myth of Marathon Monday

High-level exercisers never get heart disease.

I named this myth in honor of the elite athletes who run the Boston Marathon in my hometown every April. Many folks think that if you're fit enough to run a marathon, then you won't die of heart disease. That's an interesting concept; unfortunately, it's totally false. Every year a number of regular exercisers die of heart attacks or other acute manifestations of coronary artery disease — while they're exercising. What happened? Many forgot that coronary heart disease has multiple risk factors. An active lifestyle certainly lowers one of those risks, but you can't ignore the others. See Chapter 3 for more about risk factors.

The Myth of Pleasingly Plump

Medicalizing obesity is a subtle form of prejudice.

This subtle myth is a difficult one. As I discuss in detail in Chapter 3, obesity is an extremely significant risk for heart disease. Recently, a movement has arisen in the United States promoting "fat acceptance." The movement's basic belief is that overweight people are routinely discriminated against in the U.S. in unfortunate ways. I don't disagree, but some proponents also say that medicalizing obesity, by calling it a chronic disease, simply extends this prejudice into the medical profession. Prejudice against people who are overweight should not be tolerated by anyone, and this particularly holds true for those in the medical field. By the same token, stating clearly and unequivocally that obesity is hazardous to your cardiovascular health is a necessity. All physicians need to carefully counsel obese people about ways to lose weight and practice lifelong, healthy weight management to lower their risks of cardiovascular disease. You can look great, and you're certainly a person of great value even if you are overweight — but as for your heart, there is no such thing as being "pleasingly plump."

The Cave Man Myth

If you're having chest pain, the best thing you can do is wait and see whether it goes away.

The *Peanuts* character Linus once asked Charlie Brown how he approached a problem. Did he tackle it right away, or think about it first? Charlie Brown responded, "I try to go into a cave and hope that it will go away." That may work in other areas of your life, but ignoring the symptoms of acute heart disease is a bad idea. The longer the delay before treatment of a heart attack begins, the greater the potential heart damage. If you're having significant chest discomfort, shortness of breath, or any other symptoms that suggest a heart attack, call 911 immediately so you can be transported to the emergency room. Don't hide in a cave! See Chapter 5 for more about heart attacks.

The Myth of the Stiff Upper Lip

Dying of a broken heart or being scared to death is not possible.

Folk wisdom long has suggested that people can be scared to death or die of a broken heart. Many cardiologists, however, say that your emotions and mental state can affect your behavior but not your heart. From this point of view, it doesn't matter whether you keep a stiff upper lip and bury your fears, pain, and stress or deal with them. Yet as I discuss in Chapter 22, multiple scientific studies show that important mind/body connections exist for health in general and cardiovascular health in particular. Your levels of stress, your connection to other people, your sense of giving and receiving love all are extremely important for your cardiovascular health. Your goal should be using these profound linkages to promote cardiovascular health.

The Myth of Jupiter

We all will die of heart disease, if we live long enough.

Jupiter, the Roman King of the Gods, killed mere mortals by hurling thunderbolts from the sky. This myth expresses the presumption that heart disease is an act of God. Not so. Dying of heart disease is not inevitable. Recognize that your own habits and actions play the biggest roles in whether you develop heart disease. Let's take a tip from baseball great Mickey Mantle, who humorously said of his health-destructive lifestyle, "If I knew I was going to live so long, I would have taken better care of myself!" I don't know about you, but when Jupiter hurls those thunderbolts at me, I intend to step aside! And to do it, I'm using all the information I've shared with you here in *Heart Disease For Dummies.*

Chapter 25

Ten Great Heart-Healthy Foods

A *hearty* meal often is the way to reach your heart, isn't it? You can affirm the pleasures of the table (no food cops!) and, at the same time, adopt a balanced, moderate approach to nutrition that enhances your heart health. Chapter 20 shows you exactly how to do it. Then you can use these ten great heart-healthy foods to fine-tune your nutritional plan for improved cardiac health.

Olive Oil

Olive oil and other monounsaturated fats have enhanced the tasty food and heart health of Mediterranean people for centuries. Monounsaturated fats offer the dual advantage of raising HDL (good cholesterol) without raising total cholesterol. Of note, the American Diabetes Association also recognizes the value of monounsaturated fat and recommends that diabetics increase their consumption of it. Besides olive oil, other sources of monounsaturated fats include olives, fish, sesame seeds, avocados, peanuts, walnuts, pecans, and some other oils (peanut, walnut, canola, and sesame). The drawback? Like all oil, olive oil has 120 calories per tablespoon. So don't go wild.

Fish

I love fish! Both as a cardiologist and a food lover. Studies show substituting fish for red meat significantly lowers the amount of saturated fat in your diet and has a positive effect on lowering cholesterol levels and the risk of heart disease. This benefit is thought to be a result of the Omega 3 fatty acids in fish. Omega 3 fatty acids also lower triglycerides and may make blood platelets less sticky and thereby less likely to clot, which reduces the risk of unstable angina or an acute heart attack. Some fish, such as salmon, tuna, herring, and blue fish, are high in Omega 3 oils. But don't turn fish into a cardiac nightmare by frying it. Fish oil capsules, by the way, don't seem to provide you with the same benefit.

Soy Foods

Soy protein can help lower LDL cholesterol (the bad cholesterol) and raise HDL (the good cholesterol). Soy also contains antioxidants called *isoflavones,* which may help prevent heart disease in other ways. Although it differs from animal protein, soy protein offers a much more complete set of amino acids (the building blocks of proteins) than most vegetables, and so can be substituted for fat-rich meats. The only negatives about soy are that some people don't like its taste and that most studies suggest that you have to consume 30 to 50 grams daily to gain the cardiac benefits. (That's a lot of tofu.) But your choices are increasing as the variety of soy products grows. Using soy protein can be particularly important for *vegans* (vegetarians who eat no animal products — not even milk and eggs) for reasons beyond heart health.

Soluble Fiber

From a cardiac health point of view, I'm a soluble-fiber stalwart. Scientific evidence of soluble fiber's cholesterol-lowering benefit is so strong that the Food and Drug Administration now allows food manufacturers whose products are high in soluble fiber to state: "The consumption of soluble fiber as part of an overall low-fat diet further reduces the risk of coronary heart disease." Where can you find it? Whole oat cereals such as oatmeal or Cheerios and its clones are good. Other sources of soluble fiber include dry beans and peas, barley, whole grain oats, citrus fruits, apples, and corn. My laboratory also has done work on *psyllium,* another soluble fiber that significantly lowers cholesterol levels.

Whole Grains

In addition to soluble fiber, whole grains contain the other major type of fiber, insoluble fiber (which is very important for bulking of stools and decreasing the risk of colon cancer), as well as a variety of phytochemicals. By eating more whole grains, you can cut your risk of heart disease significantly, maybe as much as one-third or one-half. But you must make sure you're eating *whole grains,* not refined grains, which are missing valuable components, such as the husks. Unfortunately, most Americans eat less than half the recommended 25 grams of fiber every day. So what are some examples of high-fiber foods? Cereals such as oatmeal, shredded wheat, wheat germ, and bran are excellent sources of whole grains. Look for cereals that have 3 to 6 grams of fiber per serving. Whole-grain breads with at least 2 grams of fiber per serving can be another good source.

Fruits and Vegetables

Now where's my soapbox!? I simply cannot say too many good things about fruits and vegetables: Eating five servings of fruits and vegetables per day can help lower your risk of coronary artery disease, lower your blood pressure, and reduce your risk of colon cancer. They're a great source of fiber. Eating more fruits and vegetables is a great way to reduce the amount of fat in your diet. Because fresh produce now is flown in from all around the world, grocery stores are stocked year-round with high-quality, fresh produce. To encourage fruit and veggie consumption, I recommend that you keep at least three different kinds of fresh fruit available and handy — in the fridge or in a bowl on the kitchen counter or table — for easy snacking. Focus on what's in season.

Plant Sterol Esters

Plant sterol esters, or *phytosterols,* don't sound much like food, do they? But plant sterols, which help build plant cell walls, occur in all plant foods. Vegetable oils contain the highest amounts of them. Medical science has known for decades that plant sterols can lower levels of LDL cholesterol (bad cholesterol). Another plus for veggies! Recent research shows that consuming about 2 grams of plant sterol esters per day, typically in the form of plant sterol-ester-enhanced margarines, can lower LDL cholesterol from as much as 9 percent to 20 percent. If you like a little spread on your whole grain toast or bagel, you can easily make these products (such as the brands Take Control and Benecol) part of a heart-healthy diet that's high in fruits, vegetables, and fiber and low in saturated fats.

B Vitamins — Folate and B-6

Okay, so these are components of many foods. But *folate,* which is also called folic acid, and vitamin B-6 are so important that they have to make any cardiologist's top-ten list of heart-healthy food products. Both of these B vitamins help lower the blood levels of homocysteine, which at high levels has been shown to increase the risk of heart attacks. By consuming more foods containing folate and vitamin B-6–containing foods (and in some instances supplementing your diet), you can lower your risk of heart disease. Think *foliage* to help you remember what foods are rich in folate. (They have the same root word.) That means green, leafy vegetables are a good source of folate, and so are dried beans, peas, and orange juice. Fully fortified whole grain cereals and a multivitamin supplement are other sources. Good sources of vitamin B-6 include chicken, lean beef (in moderation), whole-grain cereals, and bananas, in addition to vitamin supplements.

Tea

In one of their songs, the Rolling Stones say they're just looking for "a little tea and sympathy." Well, from the cardiac standpoint, they may not be too far off. Tea, regardless of whether it contains caffeine, appears to be beneficial to the heart. Black tea is a source of *flavinoids*, which are antioxidants thought to retard the development of atherosclerosis. In one study of 700 men and women in Boston who drank one or more cups of tea per day, the risk of suffering a heart attack was less than half what it was for people who did not follow this practice.

Alcohol

Alcohol is a mixed bag for the heart. I never recommend to anyone who doesn't currently drink alcohol to start drinking it. On the other hand, a number of studies show that moderate alcohol consumption lowers the risk of heart disease. This benefit of alcohol appears to come from alcohol's ability to increase HDL cholesterol (the good form) and its ability to decrease the likelihood of abnormal clotting in the blood. Of all the forms of alcohol, red wine appears particularly beneficial because anticlotting substances and chemicals found in the skins of grapes are present longer during the wine-making process for red wine than they are in the making of white wine. These substances also are present in purple grape juice, although you need to drink about twice as much grape juice as wine to get the cardiac benefit.

A word of caution: Moderate alcohol consumption is defined as one or two glasses of wine per day, one or two beers, or one shot of distilled spirits. In the previous sentence, I want to emphasize the word *or*. Substitute the word *and* for the word *or*, and you'd reach heavy alcohol consumption — which increases your risk of heart disease, hypertension, and motor vehicle accidents.

Chapter 26

Ten Cardiac Signs and Symptoms You Need to Know About

In This Chapter

▶ Understanding which symptoms suggest heart disease

▶ Knowing when to take symptoms to the doctor

*A*lthough medical signs and symptoms can overlap, you can distinguish between the two on the basis of who is experiencing them. For example, you may regard a nagging, worrisome cough as a *symptom*. Your doctor, however, may regard that cough as a *sign* of congestion of the lungs. In broad terms, then, *symptoms* are feelings or conditions that a patient experiences and then tries to describe to his or her physician. *Signs* are findings that the physician derives from the physical examination that point toward the proper cardiac diagnosis.

Depending on the circumstances and severity, some symptoms (conditions you experience) may represent signs of serious cardiac disease to your physician or may not be worrisome at all. In this chapter, I look at ten key symptoms and signs.

Chest Pain

Chest pain probably is the most common symptom for which people go to see a cardiologist. Although chest pain can signify heart problems, it also can stem from a wide variety of structures in the chest, neck, and back that have no relation (other than proximity) to the heart. The lungs, skin, muscles, spine, and portions of the gastrointestinal tract, such as the stomach, small bowel, pancreas, and gallbladder are among these structures. Pain caused by angina or heart attack usually is located beneath the breastbone but may also be located in the front of the chest or either arm, neck, cheeks, teeth, or high in the middle of the back. Exercise, strong emotion, or stress may also provoke chest pain. Very short bouts of pain lasting five to ten seconds typically are not angina or heart-related but are more likely to be musculoskeletal pain. If you have concern about *any* chest discomfort, going to a medical facility and having it further evaluated is imperative. (See Chapters 4 and 5 for more.)

Shortness of Breath

Shortness of breath is a major cardiac symptom. But determining whether this symptom comes from problems with the heart, the lungs, or some other organ system typically is difficult. Exertion can cause temporary shortness of breath in otherwise healthy individuals who are working or exercising strenuously or in sedentary individuals who are working even moderately. But an abnormally uncomfortable awareness of breathing or difficulty breathing can be a symptom of a medical problem. Shortness of breath that occurs when you're at rest, for example, is considered a strong cardiac symptom. If shortness of breath lasts longer than five minutes after activity or occurs when you're at rest, have your doctor evaluate it.

Loss of Consciousness

Loss of consciousness usually results from reduced blood supply to the brain. Perhaps the most common loss of consciousness is what people usually call a *fainting episode.* This temporary condition may be brought on by being in a warm or constricted environment or in a highly emotional state. Such episodes often are preceded by dizziness and/or a sense of *fading to black.* When the heart is the cause, loss of consciousness typically occurs rapidly and without preceding events. Cardiac conditions ranging from rhythm disturbances to mechanical problems potentially can cause fainting or a blackout. Because such cardiac problems can be serious, never dismiss the loss of consciousness in an otherwise healthy individual as a fainting episode until that person has a complete medical workup.

Cardiovascular Collapse

You can't experience a more dramatic symptom or greater emergency than *cardiovascular collapse,* also called *sudden cardiac death.* Of course, cardiovascular collapse results in a sudden loss of consciousness, but the victim typically has no pulse and stops breathing. The victim of a seizure or fainting spell, on the other hand, has a pulse and continues breathing. Cardiovascular collapse can occur as a complication in an individual who has known heart disease but sometimes may be the first manifestation of an acute heart attack or rhythm problem. When cardiovascular collapse occurs, resuscitation must take place within a very few minutes or death inevitably follows. Being able to respond quickly to cardiovascular collapse is the greatest reason for learning CPR or basic cardiac life support. (See also Chapter 7.)

Palpitations

Palpitations, which can be defined as an unpleasant awareness of a rapid or forceful beating of the heart, may indicate anything from serious cardiac rhythm problems to nothing worrisome at all. Typically, an individual who is experiencing palpitations describes a sensation of a *skipped beat;* however, people also may describe a rapid heartbeat or a sensation of lightheadedness. Whenever the palpitation is accompanied by lightheadedness or loss of consciousness, it is imperative that a further workup be undertaken to determine whether serious, underlying heart-rhythm problems are present. Often, the simplest underlying causes of palpitations can be turned around by getting more sleep, drinking less coffee or other caffeinated beverages, decreasing alcohol consumption, or trying to reduce the amount of stress in your life. Nevertheless, you need to take this problem to your doctor for evaluation first.

Edema

Edema is an abnormal accumulation of fluid in the body, a type of swelling, and has many causes. The location and distribution of the swelling is helpful for determining what causes it. If edema occurs in the legs, it usually is characteristic of heart failure or of problems with the veins of the legs. Edema with a cardiac origin typically is *symmetric,* which means that it involves both legs. If the edema is an abnormal gathering of fluid in the lungs, called *pulmonary edema,* the typical symptom is shortness of breath. This symptom also can be typical in a patient with heart failure. Abnormal gathering of fluid in either the legs or the lungs always indicates the need for a complete cardiac workup to determine whether each of the heart's main pumping chambers is working adequately.

Cyanosis

Cyanosis, the bluish discoloration of the skin resulting from inadequate oxygen in the blood, is a sign and a symptom. One form of cyanosis occurs when unoxygenated blood that normally is pumped through the right side of the heart somehow passes into the left ventricle and is pumped out to the body. This anomaly commonly occurs in congenital abnormalities that create abnormal openings between the right and left sides of the heart. The second type of cyanosis commonly is caused by constriction of blood vessels in your limbs or peripheries and may be the result of a low output from the heart or from exposure to cold air or water. Whether the cyanosis is central or peripheral in nature guides a physician in the search for which type of underlying condition is causing the cyanosis. Any form of cyanosis is a symptom that should prompt discussion with your physician.

Cough

As anyone who has had a head cold knows, a cough can accompany a viral illness. It can also represent a variety of underlying causes such as cancers, allergies, abnormalities of the lungs, or abnormalities of the breathing tube. The cardiovascular disorders that result in cough are those that cause abnormal accumulations of fluid in the lungs, such as significant heart failure. Take any prolonged or unexplained cough to your doctor. Certainly whenever blood is present in what you cough up, you need to have the possible causes checked out. The same goes for any evidence of bacterial infection, typically yellowish, greenish, or blood-tinged sputum.

Hemoptysis

Coughing up blood of any kind — from small streaks in sputum to large quantities — is called *hemoptysis* in medicine. This condition can result from a variety of very serious diseases of the lungs or even some forms of cancer. Whatever the cause, coughing up blood-tinged secretions never is normal and may represent a medical emergency. If you ever cough up blood in any form — no matter how minor it seems — contact your doctor immediately.

Fatigue

In busy, hectic lives, *fatigue* may stem from a bewilderingly large number of underlying causes ranging from depression to side effects of drugs to physical illnesses, including cardiac problems. The ordinary fatigue you feel after working hard is normal, even when you have to crash into bed early. But a significant level of *enduring* fatigue should always prompt a call to your doctor, who may want to do an appropriate medical workup to determine possible underlying causes.

Chapter 27

Ten Secrets of Long-Term Success

In This Chapter

▶ Taking small steps for long-term change

▶ Winning the race against heart disease

*E*ffectively treating heart disease or preventing it in the first place requires making a lifelong commitment to carrying out simple heart-healthy habits and practices from day to day. Affirming the positive habits you already have and making necessary changes to nurture heart health is a race — make that an enjoyable marathon — always won by the tortoise and not the hare. In this chapter, I highlight ten key "secrets" that can make you a world champion tortoise in the marathon battle against heart disease. How can I be so sure? I've seen these strategies work for thousands of hard-shelled patients.

Educate Yourself

Former President John F. Kennedy was fond of saying, "Knowledge is power." This proverb is certainly just as true when it comes to heart disease. This entire book is dedicated to providing you with knowledge and, I hope, motivation, to discover as much as you can about those lifestyle factors and medical therapies that can lower your risk of developing heart disease or help treat established heart disease. In addition to *Heart Disease For Dummies,* many other wonderful books, periodicals, and now the Internet also can help you gather the facts that you need to be an effective partner in fighting heart disease. Don't be embarrassed or shy about bringing this information to your physician.

Accumulate, Accumulate

This particular secret applies very specifically to physical activity. Hundreds of scientific studies support the concept that accumulating physical activity in small increments throughout the day is just as effective, in terms of lowering your risk of heart disease, as establishing one period of time each day when you exercise.

But the *concept of accumulation* also applies to other aspects of combating heart disease. Each day you make hundreds of small decisions: whether to eat a piece of fruit or to have a doughnut, whether to smoke a cigarette, whether to take the elevator two flights or climb the stairs . . . you get the picture. Accumulating good decisions can make an enormous difference in long-term success in the battle against heart disease.

Be Prepared

The Boy Scouts had it right when they adopted the motto "Be prepared." Most people who have difficulty making changes in their lifestyle falter on simple issues, not profound ones. Most people ignore simple, basic preparation, making it much more difficult to accomplish changes. A good pair of walking shoes or a good all-weather exercise suit, for example, can make the difference between establishing a consistent walking program or faltering. Having the proper ingredients in your pantry makes it more likely that you'll choose something low in fat and nutritious rather than a convenience food loaded with salt and fat. Writing down your questions and being prepared to discuss side effects can make the difference between a satisfactory visit to your doctor and a frustrating one. As you see, most preparatory steps are not complex, but neglecting preparation is an invitation to frustration and failure.

Mix and Match

Variety is the spice of life — the spice of making lifestyle changes, too. Boredom sabotages the best intentions. Regardless of whether it means keeping lots of fruits and vegetables in the refrigerator to make sure that you get your requisite five a day, mapping out different walking routes, or experimenting with different forms of physical activity, adding variety can prevent things from going stale. The best way to fight boredom is to prevent it in the first place by mixing and matching to add variety to your lifestyle-change program.

Be Specific and Prioritize

Remember that most people tend to falter on simple issues, not complex ones, when making positive lifestyle changes. To accomplish any goal, but particularly ones that involve the long-term accumulation of small changes, you must be specific and prioritize. For example, each day, try to have a specific plan for how you're going to get in your physical activity. This may be as simple as establishing a time and place to walk. To stick with eating low-fat food, you can do something as simple as packing your lunch every day or always taking a piece of fruit to make sure that doughnut doesn't tempt you midmorning. Establishing a specific list of priorities also is important. Decide which changes you want to make when and take them on one at a time. Having a vague idea that you'll "get around to it" dooms you to failure.

Include Family and Friends

People are social beings. Clear evidence shows that people who connect with other human beings in positive ways and open up their hearts by sharing and loving others lower their risk of heart disease. Connecting with other people in positive ways also is a wonderful strategy for accomplishing short- and long-term goals. Bringing about changes in your life — whether it's weight management, more physical activity, better nutrition, or even smoking cessation — is much easier when you share your aspirations with family and friends. These are the people who love you most, and they want to help you. By sharing with them, you stack the deck in your favor when it comes to lifestyle changes.

Be Optimistic

Everyone has heard that an optimist sees the glass as half full, and a pessimist sees the glass as half empty. Through the years, I've become convinced that optimism is one of the greatest allies in the fight against heart disease. My patients who truly believe they're going to win the war against heart disease invariably seem to do better. Optimism is one of the reasons why I love to see patients who garden. Gardeners, in my experience, are inevitably optimistic. They plant the seeds and then are filled with hope as they tend them during the course of the growing season, watching the fruits (and vegetables!) of their labors mature to produce food and beauty. Doctors have an arsenal of many wonderful techniques and medicines in modern cardiovascular medicine, but nothing is more powerful than the human spirit in helping to control heart disease. Being diagnosed with heart disease does not mean the end of anything. It often can be the beginning of you taking charge of your life. As far as heart disease goes, attitude is everything. Strive to be an optimist.

Seize the Day

Each day, everyone faces a multitude of opportunities to choose between positive and negative lifestyle decisions. If you ask people who aren't regular exercisers why they have difficulty establishing this habit, the most common excuse you hear is "I don't have time." In the 1980s, I conducted a survey of physical activity among Fortune 500 CEOs, arguably some of the world's busiest people. Yet the average CEO was three times more likely to exercise on a regular basis than the average American adult. Clearly, these very busy individuals were making time for things that mattered to them. They were truly "seizing the day."

In my opinion, the basis for all stress reduction programs is to "seize the day." By that, I mean you need to live in the present but don't fear the future or regret the past. When it comes to lifestyle changes, people who tend to succeed are the ones who figure out how to live in the present, make the most of daily opportunities, and make positive heart-healthy lifestyle choices. They avoid the Alice-in-Wonderland Syndrome — jam yesterday, jam tomorrow, but never jam today. And of course, today's all anyone ever has. So, *carpe diem* — seize the day!

Form Partnerships

As I discuss in Chapter 12, forming a partnership with your physician and other health-care workers is one of the best strategies that you can adopt in the war against heart disease. In fact, I'm skeptical that anyone who hasn't formed such a positive partnership can truly succeed. Modern cardiovascular medicine currently relies on many wonderful techniques, medicines, and procedures, and more are being developed regularly, but your cardiologist can't help you get the most out of these techniques and procedures unless you work together as active partners. You'll find that such a partnership also can shore you up when you're tempted to backslide while making difficult lifestyle changes.

Reward Yourself

Changing your behavior is tough! When you make changes, it is therefore important to recognize that you have succeeded, so be proud of yourself and reward yourself. When you achieve any of the short-term and long-term goals you set, make a point of celebrating your success. Go out and buy yourself a new CD or treat yourself to a delicious (low-fat!) meal. Find some other positive way of marking your success. If you're living in a family with someone who's struggling to establish a positive lifestyle, make sure that you participate in celebrating and rewarding every success. Celebrate that lower cholesterol or the first-month anniversary of smoking cessation. Make a big fuss over that first ten-pound weight loss, and the next and the next. All these gestures of celebration and reward remind you that small victories lead to larger ones and that the largest victory of all is your victory over the number-one killer in the U.S. — heart disease.

Appendix

Great Heart-Healthy Recipes by America's Leading Chefs

• •

*W*hen you read the words "heart-healthy recipes" in the title above, what images flash into your mind? Dull food, tasteless as cardboard? Enough raw veggies to make you feel like a rabbit? Tiny portions of pale meat surrounded by limp, steamed vegetables? Forget those terrible images! The best heart-healthy eating, the kind you can enjoy for a lifetime, is about *good* eating, what Julia Child has called "the pleasures of the table."

If you have your doubts, these ten recipes created by top chefs prove that heart-healthy cooking can offer great taste. Think of these ten recipes as a sampler of what's possible from breakfast to dinner. Some of the recipes are simple to make; others will take a little time. All will tickle your palate. If you glance through the recipes, you'll notice that nothing — not even fat — is banished. Instead, variety and balance are emphasized. And that's in just ten recipes.

So give these a try. You can find more than 100 more recipes from these and other top chefs in *The Healthy Heart Cookbook For Dummies.* Investing a little time in exploring these recipes means finding a way of eating that's all about discovery and delicious taste, not deprivation.

Recipes in This Chapter

▶ Citrus Quinoa Salad

▶ Mizuma Salad with Oranges, Mint, and Dried Cranberries

▶ Mark's Low-Fat Oat Bran Muffins with Fresh Peaches

▶ Green Pimento and Mango Salsa

▶ Chilled Melon Soup with Anise Hyssop

▶ Grilled Maine Salmon in Lemongrass Broth

▶ Gulf Fish Court Bouillon

▶ Ratatouille (Ratatouia)

▶ Roasted Chicken with Caramelized Garlic & Sage

▶ Spicy African Chicken Soup

Citrus Quinoa Salad

Created by Alfonso Constrisciani
Executive Chef/Proprietor, Opus 251 at the Philadelphia Art Alliance and Circa
Philadelphia, Pennsylvania

Special Ingredients: *Quinoa, citrus oil (optional)*

Preparation Time: *30 minutes*

Yield: *8 servings*

For salad:

1½ cups chicken stock (vegetable stock can be substituted)

¾ cup quinoa, washed and rinsed well

¼ cup red onion, finely diced

¼ cup carrot, finely diced

¼ cup radish, finely diced

3 to 4 scallions (green onions), washed and diagonally sliced ¼-inch thick

For salad dressing:

Zest of 1 orange

¼ orange, peeled and minced

Zest of 1 lemon

¼ lemon, peeled and minced

1 tablespoon fresh lemon juice

1½ teaspoons fresh garlic, minced

1 tablespoon citrus oil or canola oil

1 tablespoon olive oil

1½ teaspoons rice wine vinegar

1 tablespoon parsley, finely chopped

Salt & freshly ground pepper, to taste

1 In a medium saucepan, bring chicken stock to a boil. Add quinoa and cook over low heat until liquid is absorbed and quinoa is tender, about 15 minutes.

2 Prep all salad vegetables while quinoa is cooking.

3 When quinoa is fully cooked, remove it from heat and strain it; then cool quinoa by spreading it out on a cookie sheet while preparing salad dressing.

4 Zest orange and lemon for dressing by finely grating outer layer of peel. Be sure to wash fruit prior to zesting.

5 Combine all salad dressing ingredients in small bowl and season with salt and pepper.

6 In a large bowl, combine all vegetables with cooled quinoa and toss with dressing. Season to taste with salt and pepper.

Nutrition Information Per Serving (based on 8 ¹/₂-cup servings)

Calories	107	Saturated Fat	0.5 grams
Protein	3 grams	Cholesterol	0 mg
Carbohydrate	14 grams	Sodium*	199 mg
Total Fat	5 grams	Dietary Fiber	2 grams

*Sodium information based on no added salt.

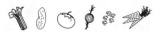

Quinoa (pronounced KEEN-wah), a grain commonly used in South American cooking, is the most protein-rich grain and contains all essential amino acids. Quinoa also is higher in mono- and polyunsaturated fats and lower in carbohydrates than other grains. Quinoa cooks like rice and expands to about twice its original volume (pasta doubles in size and rice triples). Quinoa can be purchased in many health and natural foods stores and in some supermarkets.

Mizuma Salad with Oranges, Mint, and Dried Cranberries

Created by Donna Nordin
Owner/Chef, Café Terra Cotta
Tucson and Scottsdale, Arizona

Special Ingredients: *Mizuma greens*

Preparation Time: *15 minutes*

Yield: *4 servings*

4 cups mizuma greens, washed and patted dry (can substitute mesclun salad green mix)

3 oranges

1 tablespoon fresh mint, julienned

¼ cup sweetened, dried cranberries

Salt and freshly ground black pepper, to taste

1 Fillet two of the oranges by peeling away outer rind and inner white skin. Using a sharp paring knife, cut individual sections away from the membranes that encase each section.

2 Juice the third orange. This can be done by hand. Roll the orange on the countertop, gently pressing down, for a few seconds to make it easier to juice. Then cut the orange in half and squeeze each half into a medium mixing bowl until all the juice has been released.

3 Add julienned mint and cranberries to the orange juice and mix. Season to taste with salt and pepper.

4 Add greens and toss enough to coat leaves. Arrange salad on large platter or four individual serving plates. Top with orange fillets.

Nutrition Information Per Serving (based on 8 servings)

Calories	72	Sodium*	14 mg
Protein	1.7 grams	Dietary Fiber	3 grams
Carbohydrate	17 grams	Vitamin A	24% of the Daily Value
Total Fat	0 grams	Vitamin C	88% of the Daily Value
Saturated Fat	0 grams	Folic Acid	54% of the Daily Value
Cholesterol	0 mg		

Sodium information based on no added salt. Salting to taste will significantly increase the sodium content of this dish.

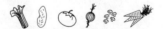

Mizuma is a delicate salad green from Japan that is often included in mesclun salad mixes. Mizuma may be found at farmer's markets or specialty produce markets during the spring and summer.

Mark's Low-Fat Oat Bran Muffins with Fresh Peaches

Created by Mark Tarbell
Executive Chef/Owner Tarbell's and Barmouche
Phoenix, Arizona

Special Ingredients: *Kosher salt (regular table salt can be substituted), 2¾ inch muffin pan*

Preparation Time: *30 minutes*

Yield: *12 muffins*

2 cups oat bran

2 teaspoons baking powder

1 teaspoon cinnamon

½ teaspoon kosher salt

1 cup nonfat milk

½ cup maple syrup

2 egg whites

2 tablespoons canola oil

1 cup diced fresh peaches (can substitute strawberries or blueberries)

1 Preheat oven to 425°F.

2 Grease muffin pans with cooking spray.

3 In a large bowl, combine the oat bran, baking powder, cinnamon, and kosher salt and stir to blend.

4 In a separate bowl, whisk together the milk, maple syrup, egg whites, and canola oil. Stir in the peaches.

5 Pour the peach mixture into the dry ingredients and stir very gently, just to combine. Lumps in the batter are okay.

6 Spoon batter into the prepared muffin tins, filling about three-quarters full.

7 Bake 15 minutes or until golden brown on top.

Nutrition Information Per Serving (based on 12 servings)

Calories	117	Saturated Fat	0 grams
Protein	4 grams	Cholesterol	0 mg
Carbohydrate	24 grams	Sodium	184 mg
Total Fat	3 grams	Dietary Fiber	3 grams

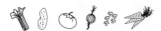

Green Pimento and Mango Salsa

Created by MaryAnn Saporito Boothroyd
Chef/Owner, Saporito's Florence Club Café
Hull, Massachusetts

Chef MaryAnn recommends serving this flavorful, fragrant, and fat-free salsa with grilled chicken or fish or baked tortilla chips. The salsa also makes a wonderful topping for baked potatoes. Don't be confused by the name of this salsa. Pimento is the Spanish term for pepper, hence the name of this salsa that combines three different peppers with fresh herbs and the sweetness of mangoes.

Preparation Time: *25 minutes*

Yield: *8 ⅓-cup servings*

2 green bell peppers	*2 tablespoons red wine vinegar*
1½ cups ripe fresh mango, peeled and diced	*2 tablespoons fresh cilantro, chopped*
½ cup red bell pepper, diced	*2 tablespoons fresh basil, chopped*
¼ to ½ cup diced hot pickled cherry peppers (Italian style in vinegar, not oil)	*Salt, to taste (analysis based on ¼ teaspoon salt)*
½ cup pineapple juice	*Freshly ground black pepper, to taste*

1 Halve and seed green peppers. Arrange the pepper halves on a baking sheet, skin side up, and place under broiler for 3 to 4 minutes until skin blisters and blackens; rotate the pan if necessary for even cooking.

2 Place roasted pepper into a bag and close it (or into a bowl and cover tightly with plastic wrap). Set aside for 10 minutes to loosen skins.

3 Peel pepper halves, discard skins, and dice. Use ½ cup for this recipe.

4 Combine all ingredients in glass bowl and let sit for at least 30 minutes.

Nutrition Information Per Serving (based on 8 ⅓-cup servings)

Calories	*50*	*Cholesterol*	*0 mg*
Protein	*0 grams*	*Sodium*	*274 mg*
Carbohydrate	*12 grams*	*Dietary Fiber*	*2 grams*
Total Fat	*0 grams*	*Vitamin A*	*34% of the Daily Value*
Saturated Fat	*0 grams*	*Vitamin C*	*58% of the Daily Value*

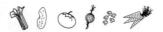

Chilled Melon Soup with Anise Hyssop

Created by Frank McClelland
Executive Chef/Owner, L'Espalier
Boston, Massachusetts

This recipe is especially appealing for an elegant weekend brunch. It calls for anise hyssop, which is an herb within the mint family that has a bitter, licorice flavor. Fresh anise hyssop may be found at farmers' markets and specialty food shops. If you're unable to find anise hyssop, you may want to try a different fresh mint. A lemon mint would give the recipe a different flavor — less distinctive perhaps — but still interesting and refreshing.

Tools: *Blender, shredder*

Preparation time: *10 minutes to prepare, 30 minutes to chill*

Cooking time: *none*

Yield: *6 servings*

2 ripe cantaloupes

2 cups Champagne or sparkling wine

1 tablespoon sugar

1 ounce anise hyssop leaves, for garnish

1 teaspoon salt

1 Peel and seed one of the cantaloupes. Cut into 1-inch chunks and place in blender with the Champagne and sugar. Blend for 1 minute. Strain; chill for 30 minutes.

2 Cut the second melon in half and seed.

3 Take a spoon and shave out the meat of the melon in thin ribbons and divide evenly among six chilled bowls. Refrigerate until ready to serve.

4 Ladle the blended chilled soup over the melon ribbons.

5 Wash anise hyssop leaves, cut into thin slices, and sprinkle on soup for garnish.

Nutrition Information Per Serving (based on 6 servings)

Calories	128	Cholesterol	0 mg
Protein	0 grams	Sodium	404 mg
Carbohydrate	19 grams	Dietary Fiber	2 grams
Total Fat	0 grams	Vitamin A	119% of the Daily Value
Saturated Fat	0 grams	Vitamin C	129% of the Daily Value

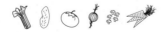

Grilled Maine Salmon in Lemongrass Broth

Created by Nora Pouillon
Chef/Owner, Nora — the only certified organic restaurant in the United States
Washington, D.C.

Special Ingredients: *Lemongrass, nuoc mam*

Preparation Time: *20 minutes*

Yield: *4 servings*

4 ounces Pad Thai noodles or rice sticks

3-inch piece of ginger, peeled and sliced

1 stalk lemongrass, outer leaves removed and thinly sliced

1 to 2 jalapeño chiles or to taste

6 cups water

2 tablespoons nuoc mam (Thai fish sauce)

2 large carrots, about 6 ounces, peeled and thinly sliced

16 shiitake mushrooms, washed, stemmed, and quartered

4 green onions, trimmed and sliced thinly on the diagonal

4 ounces watercress, stems trimmed

4 6-ounce salmon fillets, skinned

1 teaspoon canola oil

½ cup cilantro leaves, for garnish

1 Preheat your grill or broiler.

2 Soak the Pad Thai noodles or rice sticks in hot tap water for about 3 minutes or until softened. Drain and set aside.

3 Put the ginger, lemongrass, and chiles in a small chopper or food processor and process until minced, or mince finely by hand.

4 In a medium saucepan, bring the water to a boil and add the ginger, lemongrass, and chiles. Season to taste with nuoc mam. Add the carrots, shiitake mushrooms, green onions, and the drained noodles. Simmer about one minute.

5 The broth can be made ahead to this point. (If you do make it ahead, wait to add the noodles to the broth.) Just before serving, stir in the watercress. Doing so keeps it green and crisp.

6 Brush the salmon with the oil and cook about 3 minutes per side or until the fish turns opaque and medium rare.

7 To assemble, ladle the broth into four large soup bowls, dividing the vegetables and noodles evenly. Top with the salmon and garnish with cilantro.

Nutrition Information Per Serving (based on 4 servings)

Calories	308	Cholesterol	88 mg
Protein	37 grams	Sodium	854 mg
Carbohydrate	23 grams	Dietary Fiber	3 grams
Total Fat	7 grams	Vitamin A	275% of the Daily Value
Saturated Fat	1 gram	Vitamin C	79% of the Daily Value

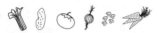

Lemongrass, with its scallion-like base, adds a sour-lemon flavor, making it a must in Thai cooking. Typically only the tender white part of the stalk is sliced or diced for use in dishes. Use the tougher tops in stock.

Lemongrass is available in Asian markets, specialty stores, and some supermarkets. No worries though if you can't find it in your local market; green onions (scallions) and a touch of lemon juice will do.

Nuoc mam is a fish sauce. When nuoc mam is combined with red chiles, garlic, lime juice, ginger, scallions, and sugar, the popular Vietnamese condiment **nuoc cham** is created. You can find nuoc mam in Asian markets and specialty markets.

Pad Thai noodles, or **rice sticks,** are a type of pasta made from rice flour that is available in Asian markets and many supermarkets.

Gulf Fish Court Bouillon

Created by Carl Walker
Executive Chef, Brennan's
Houston, Texas

Special Equipment: *Heavy-duty 18-inch aluminum foil*

Special Ingredients: *Creole seafood seasoning, Louisiana hot sauce, crab boil liquid*

Preparation Time: *60 minutes*

Yield: *2 servings*

½ cup roasted red, green, and yellow peppers, julienne cut

¾ cup tomatoes, peeled, seeded, and julienne cut

⅓ cup yellow onions, julienne cut

2 small garlic cloves, shaved thin

⅓ cup celery, cut thin diagonally

½ teaspoon Louisiana hot sauce

½ teaspoon Worcestershire sauce

2 tablespoons red wine

Couple of drops crab boil liquid

2 to 4 bay leaves

¼ teaspoon salt

⅛ teaspoon black pepper (finely ground)

2 lemon wedges

2 5-ounce fillets of red snapper (no skin or bones)

6 shrimp 16/20 count (peeled & deveined)

2 to 3 teaspoons Creole seafood seasoning

1 Arrange rack so that it sits 3 to 4 inches under the broiler. Preheat broiler. Preheat oven to 350°F.

2 Clean, seed, and halve peppers. Place the pepper halves onto a baking sheet or pan, skin side up, and place under broiler for 3 to 5 minutes until skin blisters or blackens; rotate pan if necessary for even cooking. Place the peppers into a bag and close it, or into a bowl and cover tightly with plastic wrap. Set aside for 10 minutes to loosen skins. Peel skins off and julienne flesh.

3 In a glass or stainless bowl, mix peppers, tomatoes, onions, garlic, celery, hot sauce, Worcestershire sauce, red wine, crab boil, bay leaves, salt, pepper, and lemon wedges. Set aside.

4 Take a sheet of heavy-duty 18 inch aluminum foil and lay out flat on a table. The diameter of the foil should be approximately 18 inches x 18 inches for two servings.

5 Season the fish and shrimp with Creole seasoning; then place both fillets on the aluminum foil. Place 3 shrimp on top of each fish fillet. Spoon a generous amount of the vegetable mixture on top of the fish and shrimp and cover with another sheet of foil. Fold the edges of the foil tightly 2 to 3 times on each side. Then fold each corner of the foil to create a small triangle shape. Doing so helps lock in more heat for the cooking process. *Note:* This dish can be made in a casserole dish with a cover.

6 Place the foil package on a cookie sheet and bake for 20 minutes.

7 The foil will puff up when the bouillon has finished cooking. Carefully cut around the edges of the foil and spoon into a bowl or plate. Serve with your favorite starchy side dish.

Nutrition Information Per Serving (based on 2 servings)

Calories	231	Cholesterol	84 mg
Protein	36 grams	Sodium	493 mg
Carbohydrate	11 grams	Dietary Fiber	3 grams
Total Fat	4 grams	Vitamin A	21% of the Daily Value
Saturated Fat	1 gram	Vitamin C	92% of the Daily Value

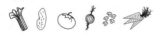

Ratatouille (Ratatouia)

Created by Constantin "Chris" Kerageorgiou
Executive Chef, La Provence Restaurant
New Orleans, Louisiana

Special Ingredients: *Coriander seeds*

Preparation Time: *2 hours*

Yield: *4 to 6 servings*

2 tablespoons plus 1 teaspoon olive oil

2 large onions, sliced

6 large garlic cloves, 4 sliced or minced, 2 put through a press or pureed

1 large red bell pepper, cut into slices about 1 inch thick by 2 inches long

1 large green bell pepper, cut into slices about 1 inch thick by 2 inches long

Coarse sea salt to taste

1½ pounds (3 medium-size) zucchini, cut in half lengthwise and sliced ½ inch thick

2 pounds (3 to 4 small) eggplant, ends trimmed, and cut into cubes

4 large or 6 medium-size tomatoes, peeled, seeded, and coarsely chopped

1 tablespoon tomato paste

1 bay leaf

2 teaspoons fresh thyme leaves or 1 teaspoon crushed dried thyme

2 teaspoons chopped fresh oregano or 1 teaspoon crushed dried oregano

½ teaspoon crushed coriander seeds

1 Heat the olive oil in a large heavy-bottomed skillet. Add the onions, garlic, and peppers, season with sea salt, and sauté over medium-high heat for 5 minutes, stirring.

2 Add the zucchini and cook another 2 minutes. Stir in the remaining ingredients and bring to a simmer.

3 Transfer the sautéed vegetables and herb mixture to a large earthenware dish and bake in a 300°F oven for 1½ hours. Check periodically, adding ¼ cup of water here and there to keep ratatouille moist.

Nutrition Information Per Serving (based on 6 servings)

Calories	171	Sodium*	30 mg
Protein	5 grams	Dietary Fiber	9 grams
Carbohydrate	28 grams	Vitamin A	32% of the Daily Value
Total Fat	6 grams	Vitamin C	207% of the Daily Value
Saturated Fat	1 gram	Folic Acid	24% of the Daily Value
Cholesterol	0 mg		

Sodium nutrition information based on no added salt. If salt is added to taste, sodium content will increase.

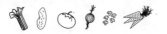

Roasted Chicken with Caramelized Garlic & Sage

Created by Walter Pisano
Executive Chef, Tulio Ristorante
Seattle, Washington

Shocking! A recipe with chicken skin in a heart-health book? Don't despair — although I'd never recommend eating poultry skin, I certainly don't discourage cooking poultry with the skin on to trap in juices. Doing so does not significantly affect the fat content of the meat but does significantly affect the final flavor. This recipe calls for caramelized garlic and sage tucked under the skin before roasting — talk about flavor!

Preparation Time: *45 minutes*

Yield: *8 servings*

4 cloves garlic (peeled)

¼ cup sugar

2 to 3 fresh sage leaves, chopped

½ tablespoon unsalted butter

4 large, whole, skin-on chicken breasts (bone-in or boneless), halved

2 tablespoons olive oil

Salt and freshly ground pepper, to taste

1 Preheat oven to 375°F. Peel and slice the garlic paper thin, and then blanch in boiling water for 1 minute.

2 Heat the sugar in a small, heavy saucepan over medium heat until golden brown. Remove from heat and add the blanched garlic, chopped sage, and butter. Mix well and set aside to cool.

3 Prepare each chicken breast by carefully pulling up the skin in one corner, at the thickest point. Slip approximately ½ teaspoon of the caramelized garlic and sage mixture under the skin. Carefully spread it around, keeping the skin attached to the meat as much as possible. You'll have extra caramelized garlic and sage, which you can use later or brush on the chicken *after* searing and before baking.

4 Season chicken with salt (optional) and pepper to taste. Heat the olive oil in a large, oven-safe skillet. (If you don't have one, you can transfer the chicken breasts to a baking dish later.) Sear each breast, skin side down, and cook over medium-high heat until skin is browned, about 5 minutes. Turn the breasts over and spread the remaining garlic/sage mixture over the browned tops, if desired.

5 Transfer the breasts in the oven-proof skillet (or in a baking dish) to the oven. Roast for 15 to 20 minutes, or until cooked through. When done, allow chicken to rest 4 to 5 minutes before removing skin, slicing, and serving.

Nutrition Information Per Serving (based on 8 servings)

Calories	181	Saturated Fat	1 gram
Protein	30 grams	Cholesterol	84 mg
Carbohydrate	2 grams	Sodium	76 mg
Total Fat	5 grams	Dietary Fiber	0 grams

Spicy African Chicken Soup

Created by Garrett Cho
Executive Chef, Palomino Euro Bistro
Minneapolis, Minnesota

Special Ingredients: *Bulgur wheat, cinnamon sticks*

Preparation Time: *2 hours (mostly simmering time)*

Yield: *16 1-cup servings*

2 tablespoons olive oil

1½ cups diced onion

1 cup chopped celery

5 teaspoons minced garlic

8 cups (64 fluid ounces) chicken stock

3½ cups (28 fluid ounces) canned tomatoes, diced, with juice

½ cup + 1 tablespoon minced parsley

½ cinnamon stick

Pinch ground cloves (about ¼ teaspoon)

2 bay leaves

Pinch cayenne pepper (about ¼ teaspoon)

2 cups uncooked bulgur wheat

12 ounces chicken breast, cut into strips approximately 1½ inches long and ½ inch thick

2 teaspoons salt (omit if using chicken broth with sodium)

1 teaspoon coarsely ground black pepper (use more to add spiciness)

1 In a large saucepan, heat olive oil over low heat. Add onions, celery, and garlic and cook, stirring often, until soft.

2 Add chicken stock, tomatoes, parsley, cinnamon stick, cloves, bay leaves, and cayenne pepper. Increase heat to bring soup to a slow boil.

3 Reduce the heat to low; simmer for 20 minutes, stirring occasionally.

4 Add the bulgur wheat and the chicken and continue to simmer for 15 minutes.

5 Remove cinnamon stick and bay leaves. Season to taste with salt and pepper.

6 Ladle soup into soup bowls. Top with unsalted, dry roasted peanuts (optional).

7 Extra soup may be frozen for 2 months or kept in the refrigerator three to 4 days at most.

Nutrition Information Per Serving (based on 16 one-cup servings)

Calories	111	Cholesterol	13 mg
Protein	9 grams	Sodium	620 mg
Carbohydrate	12 grams	Dietary Fiber	3 grams
Total Fat	3 grams	Vitamin A	23% of the Daily Value
Saturated Fat	0.7 grams	Vitamin C	21% of the Daily Value

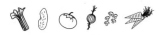

Index

• F •

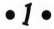

• S •

Notes

Notes